LET'S SHOP IN OUR OWN CLOSET

How to build a capsule wardrobe and find your style

Alaya Aifel

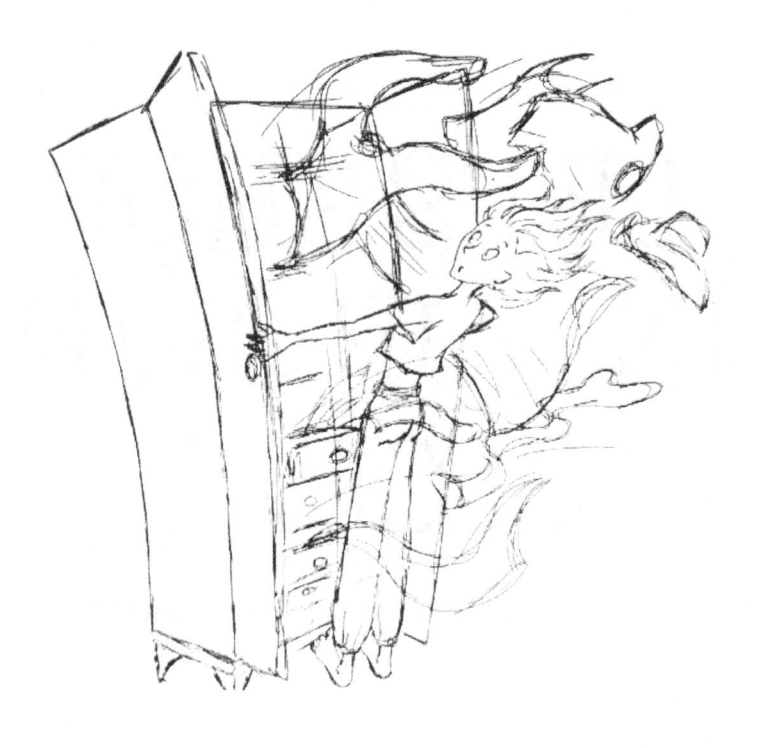

Copyright © 2022 by Alaya Aifel

All rights reserved.

LET'S SHOP IN OUR OWN CLOSET

No portion of this book may be reproduced in any form without written permission from the publisher or author, except as permitted by U.S. copyright law.

Dedications

To Vincent. Thank you for your patience

To the finest, most tactful and creative editor,
Natasha Liberman. Thank you for working with me.

Contents

1. The Most Important Chapter — 1
2. How I Created a Mini Capsule — 12
3. My Experiment — 14
4. Straight From the Hip. Step #1 Situational Wardrobe — 19
5. Step #2 How to Find Your Style While Staying Right by Your Closet — 22
6. Step#3 Skeletons in Your Closet — 26
7. Step#4 Meditative: Scale and Proportions — 34
8. Step#5 Wardrobe Structure — 38
9. Step#6 The Basics — 40
10. Step#7 Color — 47
11. Step#8 Capsule Wardrobe — 50
12. Step#9 On importance of Footwear and Bags — 55
13. Step#10 Business and Casual domain — 62
14. Step#11 Building capsule — 65
15. Step#12 Concept and Vizualization — 88
16. Step#13 Summing up — 92

17. Step #14 How to Part with Clothes   98
18. Step #15 Conclusion and Some Reflections about Styles   102
19. Finding your Style   106
20. How to Find Your Style "Inside-Out"   108
21. How to Find your style "Ouside-In"   111
22. Suzanne Caygill's Seasonal Color Analysis   114
23. Winter Color Type   116
24. Spring and Summer Color Types   120
25. Fall Color Type   126
26. On branding and color palette   129
27. Your expectations from the book   136

Thank you   138

Chapter One
The Most Important Chapter

Hello!

I am so glad you are here! It means you have made a decision. You are not quite sure what it is you've decided yet, but you are curious. Get your favorite drink, make yourself comfortable, and let's get started.

Let me introduce myself.

I am a woman who has risen from the hell of shapeless knitwear.

The reasons I ended up in this particular hell were not only personal, but also embedded in my ignorance of styles. One of my tasks here is to talk you out of buying faded, too close-fitting, outdated, weak, or weight-adding clothes. However hard you work on colors or proportions, if your closet is full of clothes like that, no good will come of it. Unfortunately, every brand still offers out-of-date fashions, from expensive to affordable.

There is nothing unique or original in my story. For a long time I lived extrinsically. Of course, it caught up with me! I mean the existential crisis, may it never rest. Style and clothes are not truly psychological, but they're awfully close. My resurrection came about just as fast as one restores the Feng Shui order in a closet – that is very, very slowly. But I did manage it in the end. As we talk, I'll share my sartorial stories with you and you might recognize yourself in some of them.

There may be a great many reasons for the wardrobe problem, but this is what the symptoms look like.

1. Torture. Every time you are invited to go out or visit someone, there it is. You are tormented by trying to build a look and the result is that you wear the same things over and over again. The change of seasons may be quite an agony for some people too. It's because you have just pulled through and adapted to one, just barely put together a couple of looks, and wham! Here comes spring. You've nothing against spring; you were even waiting for it. But now you have to go through the whole painful process again and come up with some other outfits. The worst case scenario is when you simply don't go out because "there is nothing to wear," although you have quite a lot of clothes. All in all, your closet is full and happy, but you feel very lonely.

2. You are shy, thinking that style is only for the slim and fit in order to make them even more perfect.

These, I think, are in a minority. The rest of us realize that style is a friend to regular women who laugh a lot and are dappled with expression lines; who swell up in the mornings and see red streaks on their face; who have no stamina for a healthy diet, lymphatic drainage exercises, jogging, or Pilates.

3. The time spent by the closet irritates you. You are one of those people who want to spend their brainpower on crypto currencies or on planting tomatoes, while looking first-rate. Well, it's a good and healthy ambition. I'm with you there.

4. You have become environmentally concerned. The army of planet-defenders is your best friend. You are top-rate at clearing space, but have no idea what to do with all that emptiness.

5. Somewhere deep down, you feel that it is much more convenient not to change anything; it is easier to simply complain about life and leave everything as it is. So you are in denial and your brain conveniently provides a very convincing idea that "you can't solve the wardrobe problem without money."

6. You may be spontaneous. You go shopping, and it seems you had a list when you started, but, somehow or other, it just got away from you. What you'd really like is a minimalistic wardrobe that is actually pretty.

Personally, I was close to problems number one and six. Shopping did not produce beauty for me and I kept doing it over and over. I kept hitting the same button, so the money just kept pouring away. The best thing was – I never gave up! I kept running after yet another top, even though the result was exactly nil.

Yes, most people do just that. Chaos in the closet is the springboard to good appearance. The closet disappoints, but it also gets you ready for the idea that you really do have to study the laws of style. It is hard, it's almost unbearable, but it's got to be done. There are classes. Even though, in the end, they scare you off even worse. After all, they make you rob yourself of an enormous amount of time, and not just yourself, but your family and all the things you love to do, simply to work out what style is.

That is why, sometimes, you can trust someone else. Me, for example. You don't know me; it is unclear why you should listen to me, but I have studied all aspects of fighting chaos in the closet for nine years. Of all the reasons listed, I have the closest relationship with reason number three. Until recently, reasons number one and six were quite important too. I worked out all the ins and outs of taming an unruly wardrobe and now I inspire people to build capsules.

Going to a stylist is a good solution, but it's like tossing a coin: you might become prettier or just poorer; will your tastes be compatible? Investing in your own knowledge, on the other hand, is forever. So, those of you who want to solve their wardrobe problem – just keep reading.

First, let me tell you a truth. Solving the wardrobe problem requires some minimal strategy at the very beginning. It's not hard; it's actually fun. You have to decide, right now, to become stylish. Not just clean up your closet to get a breathing space, not simply find some clothes to cover your body, nor make a feeble attempt at becoming prettier, but to become a truly stylish mistress of your wardrobe and, let's think on a grand scale here, become the true mistress of your life!

Your first investment is a few dollars you paid for this book. That's all, for now. Your key tools in conquering the world are YOU and your closet. We'll analyze your wardrobe to the fullest extent, so that every element works to give you beauty and good vibes.

Now, it's time to be surprised. The first stage in preparing to be stylish is over.

My dear ladies, this is the where the fun begins!

You may have heard or read in various blogs or magazines about trends, about what you should and shouldn't wear. Actually, ANYTHING WORKS. The fashion is so generous that it gives us versatility. That's because societies differ. There are people who only wear torn jeans. Then, there are those who only wear gowns. And then, there are people who wear jeans, gowns, and overalls and yet, there are those who use EVERYTHING.

We live in amazing times when nearly everything is in fashion. You choose what it is that you will choose. What works best? What is most comfortable? Where do you feel in your element? That's where you start. You can add on everything else a bit at a time or selectively.

Let me tell you where I stand: you can look gorgeous even in a basic wardrobe and not bother studying any other styles. That is what this book is about: how to build an exciting and self-sufficient basic wardrobe. Don't get hung up on the word 'basic', though. It's not at all what you think. Please get rid of anything you know about styles and keep a completely open mind for what I'll tell you.

So, stop getting worried over trends and over the fact that they changed while you blinked and you need to buy something new again. What you need to do is systematically put together the wardrobe that comes to you the easiest.

You need to realize that alarming the customers (that is us) is the classic way to manage us. Everyone and everything keeps telling us that we need to be successful, well-groomed, confident, healthy, up-to-date, efficient, fit, stylish, sophisticated, rich, or the best version of something or other, even though yesterday (and five years ago) we were just fine. Social media keeps telling us that we have to keep climbing up or we'll be just like everyone else. So, all of us (the everyone else) are just standing there staring at each other in dismay because there is so much to do, but there is no confidence, perfection, temperament, money, or pep. After all, there are still the kids, everyday life, obligations...

This kind of worry is paralyzing and the person does nothing at all. They simply worry and don't do anything. But it would be so wonderful to be beautiful. You can really go crazy that way and start hating fashion and successful fashionistas.

Don't.

There is a simple plan that works.

Don't let this storm of advertising carry you away. At this stage, the goal is to build our first capsule. I don't know WHAT you should wear. I know HOW to build a capsule.

It may be that taking a definitive step into a capsule is not your goal and you are wondering whether it's worth it.

The answer is categorical, "It is!"

Putting together a capsule and being thrilled by it is quite like implementing human design in real life. It's just as powerful. Alright, if you don't like power metaphors, then putting together a capsule and being thrilled by it is quite like learning Italian. Imagine how you exchange sweet nothings with a handsome barista in Florence. You are stretching happily like a cat that's had plenty of cream and your colleague is giving a crooked smile as they look at the two of you

What is a capsule? It's a miniature wardrobe, collected for a certain purpose, where your clothes, just like a good basketball team, seamlessly play with each other. Actually, anyone can collect twelve pieces of clothing. But getting them to reflect your personal style and work with each other is a bit more complicated.

There's one more thing. If you really want to become the mistress of your wardrobe, you have to love yourself and your closet with everything that's in it. You also have to make up your mind to build your first capsule. It might not turn out perfect, but if you get the blues every time you stop by your closet, your first capsule will be a breakthrough, a bridge to a new life.

We'll discuss only the important things, but we'll start with something easy and then keep going deeper and deeper.

Speaking of depths, back at the very beginning I did not mention quite an interesting problem.

Let us say that there is a lady who graduated from MIT, and did her PhD at Princeton, and has a whole bunch of other achievements under her belt, but she still looks like a tired sixth-grader. Her clothes do not broadcast either her intellectual abilities or her sophisticated inner world. Here's another example: a different lady this time, who is tired of being strong and independent, her heart is yearning for sympathy, but she dresses just like a warhorse. She would like her inner flower to be appreciated but she dresses like a charger ready for battle. (I want to make a reservation here: all characters are fictional, I have nothing against either MIT or Princeton; so if you recognize yourself in any of the descriptions – it is just a random coincidence). This last example is part of the same story. You open your closet and you don't like nearly everything that is in it. You wear the clothes, but you don't respect them.

You have no idea how many works there are on this subject, how many books, classes, videos, webinars, and articles have been written and made. Yet, nothing much has changed. The subject is essential; it is vital and fundamental, yet it still gets a lot of people down. Every time I tried writing about it, I would have my tenth cup of tea, go for a walk, or do something nice instead, simply in order to avoid it.

While you're ruminating on all this, I'll tell you an interesting fact about will power. It turns out that only one out of every fifteen people reaches the goals they set for themselves. The rest give up in a few days or months. Did you know that? If you are that one out of fifteen with strong will power, go on to the next chapter. If you're not, hang on for a bit longer here.

It seems that in order to go on to a gluten-free diet or to start jogging in the mornings it is not nearly enough to just do it. First, your internal parliament has to approve the new bill. That's because jogging in the morning means you lose an hour of sleep, which is a crime against humanity. Switching to a gluten-free diet means never having croissants again and that's a crime too. To make any significant changes in yourself, you have to 'ripen' for them. Sometimes, people take months to ripen. After all, important things are at stake here. Sometimes, your body even has to change your endocrine profile. To 'ripen' means to enter into negotiations with your body and promise it something that is truly more delicious than croissants or to compensate the lack of sleep with something so nice that all you have left is the ardent desire to jog in the morning.

A couple of pages earlier you decided to be the absolute mistress of your wardrobe. How did you make that decision? Let me guess: you said something like, "Yeah, yeah, I've heard that a hundred times, I'll just keep reading."

Many people think that evolution of the wardrobe is not as nearly as painful as doing abs exercises. And do you know why?

It's because the solution seems so simple. What, I? With my two degrees? I can't figure out clothes? But this simplicity is misleading. Otherwise, you would never have opened this book, there would be tons of beautifully dressed people out there, and much, much fewer clothes would make their way to the second-hand stores or even trash cans.

While you are ripening and negotiating with yourself, I will list all the goodies you can expect if you win. I don't know if my arguments will help your internal parliament to make the right decision, but I am an optimist.

- You'll spend less on clothes and can save some money for other things.

Save money for what? For going out to a really nice restaurant or for going away for a weekend, for example. Look for things that make your body sing and purr;

- You will be a beautiful, energetic, rightful mistress of your wardrobe.

This statement may seem as cheap as poor-quality knitwear. What it actually means is feeling like a tigress right before she springs. Give the feeling of beauty to your body and enter that state as often as you can. It feels great! To drive the point home, you can hum "Teach me tiger…" I've a feeling that if you can get into that state often, the wardrobe problem won't be the only one you solve;

- You will create good Feng Shui in your closet and stop wasting brainpower every morning.

It's like an army boot camp: you'll be able to get up and get dressed while a match is burning. So there you are, half asleep and at work. You have your first cup of coffee and get your blood going. Your eye falls on your reflection and you see a beauty! And she's dressed marvelously! And she's you! If you can afford the luxury of an unhurried morning, then it works differently. After morning ablutions and meditation, you open your closet and see lots of air and space and clothes that are your friends. You get dressed, take a selfie and quietly enjoy yourself. Or you can enjoy yourself out loud by sharing it on Instagram.

- You will make your contribution to the future. That way you can make sure that your grandchildren and great-grandchildren have an idea of what a clean river or a real tree looks like; as well as admire a beautifully dressed grandma. Putting your closet in order is just like building a smart home that not only makes your life safer and more comfortable, but also reduces your expenses and takes care of the environment. You will build your smart wardrobe, consuming less and getting more joy out of it.

What? You're not a grandma and not even a mom yet? You're not planning on having children at all? Hold on, don't get distracted here. Maybe I didn't say it right. I am talking about fresh air by a clean river and a feeling of personal involvement in creating beauty.

- You will advance in understanding yourself and your personal style.

What is more intoxicating than wine? Rudyard Kipling says that it's women, horses, power, and war, but I say that it's the ecstasy of discovery. The discovery, for example, that a new shirt turns your cheeks into peaches or that a sweater can embrace you just as tenderly as your loved one.

- You will become the reason, not the consequences, for the circumstances of your life!

I think I'm getting carried away here. I am sorry, but the tigress-before-the-spring wants to be here too. Actually, I am talking about changing reality, about shifting your mood by using clothes. I realize that these are just broad terms. Let me give you an example.

Let us say, you have finished the book and have built your first capsule.

So, you run out to grab some doughnuts wearing deliberately chosen jeans and T-shirt from your first capsule.

You start imagining that you're a super-star and that you had several stylists work on your image, the ones who specialize in 'low key' looks. You even have paparazzi following you. I assure you, the way you walk will change and your body will try to avoid imaginary cameras.

At the store:

Instead of doughnuts, you buy spinach and ginger (you do have paparazzi watching you and you're a super-star and an ambassador of a healthy lifestyle).

At home:

On an empty stomach (thanks to the spinach and ginger) you get a brilliant idea on how to make tons of money. You put the idea to life, you become rich, and a couple of years later you hire a 'low key look' stylist. The stylist is quite expensive and comes up with just the same kind of outfit that you wore two years ago when you ran out to get some doughnuts.

This is probably what they call Spiral Dynamics.

But joking aside, I have good news for you. The longest chapter in this book is over. I had made it this way on purpose, like an outfit through which the eye needs to travel. That is so that you would come to this

Fun,

Exciting,.

Life-transforming decision!

Chapter Two
How I Created a Mini Capsule

Before starting to write this book, I had to try and build a mini-wardrobe of 16 to 20 items and live with it for a few months. My actual personal wardrobe is not large, but there are certainly more than 20 pieces of clothing in it.

I felt a lot of resistance to the idea, which disguised itself as lassitude or family cares. It seemed that I could dispense with the experiment; after all, I knew all about it. My thoughts ran around like insects on the surface of water. I believed in the idea, but I was toying with it rather than looking at it in-depth.

And then the flood came...

Our house overlooks a large creek that is officially called a river. I have dreamt of just such a house as I looked at a movie star who was bouncing around her country kitchen on a TV screen. Later on, as I was taking a shower in my dream-house-come-true, I often heard the voice of my illusory Mary Poppins, "You shouldn't watch so much TV!"

One summer, there were heavy rains everywhere within 60 miles of the house. In a few days, the water in our creek rose by nine feet and spread out to around 50 yards. Naturally, the water went through the entire ground floor of the house. Faithful to all rules of perversity, the pump that would have helped to get the water out broke the day before. That's how we ended up carrying river water in buckets from the house back to the river.

That was the first time I felt the power of the water element. And, talking of elements, I became much more aware of the energy of people with the Summer coloring. They are just as smooth and flowing as our river, but once they overflow their boundaries, watch out! Summer women can weave tapestry (I can't even imagine it!), work as senior accountants, keeping every pencil bought in their head, or write the multi-volume Harry Potter saga. And they'll do it quietly, powerfully, and mellifluously.

But I am digressing.

It was a good thing that the adrenaline lasted only 24 hours. The water went down in the night.

Then there was the exhausting clean-up. Everything that was touched by dirty water had to be dealt with. Later on, an expert came and said that the plaster had to be removed all the way to the bricks, some floors should be replaced, and the kitchen and heaters needed to be taken out. The house ought to be left to dry for a few months and only then would it make sense to repair it.

We had to clear all the damaged areas and find housing for several months.

Only those who have ever been through something like that would know how I felt.

So we moved.

Yes, I had time to pack and take everything I wanted with me, but I was tired. I was more than tired, I was exhausted. I half-heartedly packed a rough outline of a capsule.

Chapter Three

My Experiment

You can dress pain in all sorts of ways. I dressed my exhaustion in jeans.

Dawnn Karen wrote Dress Your Best Life . She is the pioneer of Fashion Psychology and she conducts surveys on relations between attire and attitude the results of which boil down to this: There are two ways of getting dressed: in Mood Enhancements or in Mood Illustrators.

We know that when we feel out of sorts, we want to wear something shapeless, something that would help us hide, get lost, or disappear altogether.

The same thing happened to me: I had to pack, carry boxes, drive my daughter to and from school; and so I chose the Mood Illustrator way.

I simply went with the flow caused by the flood. Jeans and sweaters pulled me down even further. Don't do what I did!

Try to do a shift if you're stuck.

I think this is familiar to anyone who ever broke up with a partner or quit their job. What do we always do in a crisis? We change our hair style or go to a beauty salon!

When we need to change how we feel, we dress our pain beautifully. We transform our mood through beauty (make-up, fragrance, clothes). You cannot stay depressed when you are dressed beautifully. Just like you cannot stay depressed if you change the position of your body. Many researchers have conducted studies on the subject, not just Dawnn Karen.

When a superhero takes on his or her role, they must have their second skin, their outfit. It gives them superpowers and makes them ready for action. After all, we are all superheroes in the My Life series. Who is your costume director? And how do you get ready for action?

Incredible as it may seem, you can change your life simply by changing your clothes and becoming prettier.

There are people who like routine. Could that be you?

You always wear approximately the same thing. You have a 'uniform', just like Mark Zuckerberg, and broadcast the message to the world that "I express myself through my work." You are not ready to buy 'fashion' outfits or you simply don't have the time.

In that case, you can do a mood shift simply by using make-up or changing your hair. You can use simple accessories: bracelets or pendants. Empower them. Maybe you have jewelry that came to you from your mother or grandmother? You are already connected to it. Every time you want to change how you feel, simply add it to your uniform.

But let's go back to the capsule.

It was time to move. I took with me two pairs of jeans: blue, wide ones with a high waist and black, straight ones with a lower waist. I also took two sweaters, a sweatshirt and a short hoodie. My outdoor layers were a bomber jacket and a long coat. Then there were sneakers, brogues, and a pair of boots. Oh, yes, there were also two or three T-shirts and knitted tops.

For the first couple of weeks, I went around looking like an Environmental Refugee or a Baseball Mom: jeans, sneakers, and bomber jacket. I got tired of that role very quickly. Somebody did say that it was the role that got tired not the personality. Creating many roles is the way to mental health. Not every role gets its own outfit, but still, why not look at your wardrobe from that point of view?

In a few weeks, I gave up and got myself a long A-line skirt. It looked good with the short white hoodie. Thus my life was diverted by a Suffragette. Even though the Suffragette is emancipated, she is still a woman. In addition, she wore a long coat and brogues and after the bomber jacket it felt like an ode to elegance.

The next one who asked to be let in was the Mystery Woman. She didn't need anything special: a black knitted top, jeans, and a pair of exotic earrings was all she wanted. The Mystery Woman lived in the earrings.

As soon as we got settled in the rented apartment, I ran back to the house and brought back three things: a mini-skirt, a purple sweater, and a pair of straight purple pants. This brought out the Elegant One and the Mini-skirt. They shared the same sweater with striking shoulders.

The Elegant One wore a total purple look and accessorized it with hoop earrings or a scarf. She went to visit friends or to see performances at the community theater. She lent the pants to the Environmental Refugee, so she wouldn't turn into a vegetable with all that casualness. Mini-skirt was dressed well. I mean, there were boots at the bottom and a long coat on top. She did not go out a lot, just once a month to a wine bar, but having her there made things more fun.

There should have been another a couple more to join the role lot, but they never did.

I spent four months wearing approximately 20 items, including shoes and outdoor clothes.

Before summing up my reluctant experiment, I would like to talk a bit about make-up. I am sure that most of my readers know more about make-up than I do. My personal armory is sparse: my bare face and my made-up, second face, which simply means foundation, some eye shadow, and a bit of lipstick. I am not involved in public speaking, I don't attend haute ton events; all in all, I can't boast of a great variety of drawn self-portraits.

Yet, if you like masterpiece make-up and if you already have several excellent masks, I congratulate you. You know better than I do that masks create roles and help to shift the mood.

So, what conclusions can we draw?

A capsule is like a magnifying glass. I have seen yet again my yang passion for pants, which make up seventy percent of my wardrobe. That is why I decided to take a good look at this particular side of things, review all my pant outfits, and look closely at the jeans.

I like jeans. Driver-mom, as well as Writer and Environmental Refugee played solo parts in my role theatre. That is why I wanted the jeans to be not just good, but superlative.

In a few months, the black jeans gave out. I wore them stoically, but then it got to me: who am I trying to prove things to? I can wear them for another two months, but why should I? I liked how they fitted my legs, the color was fine, the side-seams were interesting, but the look at the hips was depressing. I went to the house for the under-study. Instead of jeans, I now had suit pants of the same color. They fitted me great and I looked more elegant.

In the third month, I upgraded my sneakers. I had to. The old ones were three-years-old and torn. I got somewhat more glamorous sneakers that sparkled. I was thinking of getting two pairs of white sneakers. After all, if I spend more than half my time as Driver-mom, why not go all out for that particular look?

What else? I didn't have enough roles. I particularly missed the one that would be called Revolution. I was burning up inside. It seemed like I was losing control. What kind of life did we have! First the corona virus and quarantines and then the flood! I was tired of sleeping on the floor, I was tired of plastic furniture (the apartment we rented was unfurnished and we filled it with garden furniture)! When, when would I have the time? I had to activate my superhero. I had to have something red, complicated, and festive. Something that could play the ice-breaker across the circumstances of my life!

I also missed the Romantic One. The Suffragette simply refused to be romantic and the Mini-skirt came out too rarely. I needed the third Grace and I needed her quickly.

So that's my story.

Let's create yours now. I am inviting you to step up to your closet.

Chapter Four

Straight From the Hip. Step #1 Situational Wardrobe

L ook at your closet as if you've never seen it before. Take a step. Find the hypothetical line by the closet and step across it. This will be a symbolic act of transition into a new situation. Take a deep breath. Open the door.

Nope, there is no Narnia there.

Yet, there may be quite a lot of strange inhabitants. Are you sorry to evict the poor dears? That's right, where would they go; you can't leave them without a roof over their head! Don't worry. You must have heard a hundred times that you need to separate your clothes into three piles (throw away, wait, and stay) and you must have done it just as many times. That's not what you're here for, after all.

Let's get going gradually, a step at a time. So, your first exercise is called "situational wardrobe". Let's move the nice and serviceable, but rarely used things out of sight.

What might these things be?

Let me illustrate using my own experience.

BUSINESS

Even if you do not work in a corporation with a strict dress code, there are still special occasions. You may want to raise your level of inscrutability in a Parent-Teacher conference. Or prove to everyone that not only are your muffins the best, but you are also the most business-like of all business ladies. Or you may need to go to an interview with corporate officers, ask them about the salary, rejoice that you've been invited to an interview at all, and proudly tell them "No, I don't think this will work for me."

I have several things for those occasions. Their numbers are diminishing, but I store what's left separately.

SPORTS CLOTHES

There are sports that you do regularly. For instance, you may turn into a tango diva three times a week. At the same time, you may also have a pair of ski pants that you use to hike in winter time or roll around in the snow, but somehow, you don't treat yourself to that type of fun too often. I suggest that you move the ski pants and similar items. Where should you move them to? Maybe to the guest room, or another closet, or storage boxes in the attic. The important thing is to remember where you've put them.

WEDDING DRESSES AND EVENING GOWNS

I don't know what your life is like, but I have attended very few gala events in the last three years. If you have no room to move them, you can store these things in a dark case so that they do not create visual litter.

HERITAGE

Oftentimes, this is something embroidered. You have inherited it or one of your loved ones has put their heart into it. It may be a handkerchief, a blouse, a dress or a doily. It makes a pleasant pause when you go through your clothes. You sit down, feast your eyes on the embroidery and cannot possibly imagine what you would wear it with. The pause ends and, hoping that one day these things will sing their swan song, you put them back. Don't do it! If you can't part with them, at least, keep them somewhere else. Better yet, have a photo session and then feast your eyes on the pictures. This advice is good for anything from your past that you find hard to part with.

SUMMER CAPSULE – THE HEAT

There is no need to explain this. If you have a lot of summer and just a bit of winter, then the winter capsule will be the rare occasion. There are also summer clothes that work year-round. They can stay.

What else can come under this heading?

CLOTHES THAT ARE TOO SMALL OR TOO BIG

I believe you! I am positive that you will get to the weight you want! When that day comes, you can revive them. In the meantime, put them out of sight.

Lastly, things you wear when you paint walls or do gardening. Christmas, freak or carnival outfits, you know what your life is like better than I do.

We'll work with what's left next. You'll need a notebook. We'll take a lot of notes.

Stop right there. Please select and put away your situational wardrobe before you read on.

Chapter Five

Step #2 How to Find Your Style While Staying Right by Your Closet

What do you think you like to wear?

It's a tough question for a lot of people. Multi-million trainings are based on this question. After all, everyone wants to be understood without saying a word.

We'll do three exercises in this chapter. Most of the information on this subject is in the chapter on "How We Look for Our Style" in the second part of the book.

Let's look into your closet again.

First, let's take the outer layers off the onion: this includes things like, "I bought it because it was in my size and on sale," "My mom gave it to me," "That's my sister's hand-me-down," "This is for Instagram," "I went shopping with a friend and got carried away." Your brain will try to get around you and rationalize everything. You have to be firm about it. Here's a 50's dress that you've never worn. Your brain tells you, "So, you don't have a purse to match, you'll wear it as soon as you find one." Are you sure your dress does not belong in a museum? Where's that purse that the dress has been waiting for for five years?

Answer this one straight out: do you wear skirts? How often? I realized that 70 percent of the time I am a pants person. I turn into a skirt person in the spring. Are you sure that you like to wear jackets? How often do you wear them? What about in winter, under a coat?

Divide your clothes into the ones you love and all the rest. Hang up your truly loved clothes separately. There is no need for them to be strewn all over your closet. Put them all together.

Now that we've taken off the outer layers, we're at the heart of the matter.

What do you do if you still don't know what you love? Answer this question: If you were to have a date with James Bond tonight (just going out for coffee), what would you wear? If Bond does not make you blush, pick any other name.

Here is another helping question: If you had to leave everything and start your life with one small suitcase, what would you put in it?

Remember that you are a live, expanding organism. You are not about to sign your final verdict.

Why do you love what you love? And let's not put any Shakespearian drama into it.

Let's do one of the most interesting exercises on the subject. Take two or three things that you absolutely love, even if they include an old sweatshirt. Add to them accessories, furniture, a flower, a gadget. You have to truly love every single thing I named 200 percent and it can't be something abstract like "I love all Swarovski crystals." It should not be just "I love orchids," but "I love my orchid with snow-white petals." You might not even have the thing. Find a photo, if you don't have it. Maybe this particular Marie Antoinette-style cabinet draws you irresistibly. Art? Most likely, you can feast your eyes on the picture your daughter made in art class all your life. You can expand the list of items a little, like add a car to it, for example.

Now you need to figure out why you love what you love. Write out seven to ten adjectives that describe each item.

If you do the exercise honestly, you'll see repetitions. You will see a recurring theme in each item description. Congratulations! You now have a list of your values. Many people are surprised by the result. I was astounded. Well... I sort of knew about it, I had an idea. But when the letters all lined up and stared at me with the same look, I felt disturbed. So that's what my values look like!

Now you know what to ask yourself when you are about to buy something. Does it help you broadcast what you value?

We'll get more specific as we go on.

What themes are the same for your favorite clothes? Is it the color, the athletic style, the high-waist fit of the pants? Do you like prints or are you more into solid colors?

Everyone has a natural feeling for what suits them and what doesn't. You already know what nourishes you and gives you energy.

For example, what kinds of prints do you like in interior design or in clothes? Here's a list that may lead you in the right direction: pyramids, impressionism, cubism, polka dots, spring flowers, feathers, waterfalls, butterflies, fall leaves, lace, exotic birds, leopard prints, snowflakes, hearts, stars, drops...

What about textures? Do you prefer a smooth surface or a rough one? Sometimes, just the print on fabric gives it a texture as, for example, happens with leopard prints. That is why freckles on a smooth skin also give it some texture. You can picture this feature as a scale where on the one end there is an elderly person with deep wrinkles and wiry, fizzy hair and on the other – a person with smooth skin and silky straight hair. Do coarse knitting, fur lapels, buttons, snaps, or screws suit you?

Write down your observations and make sure to put a date, you'll be interested in looking at your notes later on.

Loosen up as you write. We're just starting!

So, what do you do with things that are not in the 'absolutely favorite' category?

Wear them. It's crystal clear what your favorites are, but the other ones need to be tested. There is a chance that some things will migrate to the favorite category and others may do just the opposite.

Oof! We're not going away from the closet. There is still work to do. I suggest that you take a break, though, and treat yourself to a cup of hot chocolate or some jasmine tea.

Chapter Six
Step#3 Skeletons in Your Closet

Let's keep working on your style report.

Let us find the skeletons in your closet, in other words, your formulas. How many do you have and how many doubles and extras are there?

Here are some examples of formulas: skinny jeans and tunics, high-waist jeans and short tops, midi skirts and jackets. You get the idea.

What are doubles? They are recurrences of the same formula. It may be that the same combination is repeated ten times and it works. Look at your favorite fashion icons like Victoria Beckham, for example. It may also be just the other way around.

Do you keep buying carrot-colored pants with a high waist? It may be a good sign or a bad one.

On the one hand, you may have found your style and are simply perfecting your formula; you keep in touch with fashion and are adapting your silhouette.

On the other hand, it may mean that you are stuck in your habits. You learned how to dress around twenty years ago and are now just keeping up the outdated flow. Do you think this may be just the right time to try something new? Karl Lagerfeld, the creative director of Chanel said that "People who say that yesterday was better than today are ultimately devaluing their own existence."

Are you stuck or have you found yourself? You are the only one who knows the answer to that.

Devise three or four key formulas for your wardrobe.

For example, one woman who was a CEO found this combination to wear to work: a pair of pants and a blouse with a round neck and no turn-back collar (it was just great that she got rid of the collar!). When she was in her office, she wore sneakers and her jacket hung on the back of a chair. If she had to go out to a meeting and impress someone, she would put on the jacket (that acts as masculine armor nowadays), wear high heels to scare them even more, and march into battle.

My two most common silhouettes are pants and a sweatshirt or a short top with a midi skirt. You'd think that's just about as dull as ditch water... Not at all! I still can't get over how versatile these seemingly boring silhouettes are.

Now let's talk about doubles. There are obvious doubles, such as same-style tees in slightly differing colors, or several pairs of the same type jeans. You decide what to do with them. As you build your capsule, you will figure out what should be included in it and what shouldn't.

There are also color doubles, implicit ones. Pay attention now! For example, you may have straight gray pants and straight gray jeans. You can argue with that and say that jeans and pants are as different as chalk and cheese. However, an outsider only sees a gray blob at the bottom. It's not really important whether they see pants or jeans. If you have truly decided to go for reducing your wardrobe and increasing its versatility, you won't get anywhere without color. We'll talk about color a lot.

In addition to doubles, there are extras. In movies, they are actors who perform in nonspeaking roles. Let's take a sweater, for example. Let's say you have several. There is your favorite, the dark blue one, which is the main character, and then there are doubles and extras. The extra sweater is not an exact copy of your favorite one. So, it is not quite a double, nor is it a color double because it's green. It doesn't play that much of a role though; all it does is substitute for the blue sweater while it's in the laundry. The extra sweater doesn't go with much of anything except jeans and doesn't bring you all that much joy; you bear with it because needs must. As soon as the blue sweater has had its rest and has been refreshed it goes right back to work because nothing can ever be a match for the prima donna.

Extras or stars-in-reserve can be more or less talented. You are the company director. It's your decision whom to fire and whom to keep.

I am sure my editor will say that I am just beating about the bush, but I will say it again (I think, the subject of doubles makes you want to repeat yourself). What formulas do you wear the most? This is important. In a sense, we are discovering the essence of what your style is today. Find the pot of gold, stop there, and zoom in.

I don't think you should start with a total makeover when you deal with style. It makes you euphoric for a while and then there is a backlash. If you love jeans, T-shirts and cardigans, consider this outfit in details. We all know that that's where the devil is. What can be done to improve it? Is it the print on the shirt, the width of the leg, the contrast, or is the look not stiff enough? Take this combination to the level of the podium (or, at least, wear it up to your personal internal throne). Here is how you do that. I suggest that you go to an on line store, such as Sacks Fifth Avenue, Pret-a-Porter or Farfetch and find a look with items like yours: jeans, a cardigan, and a T-shirt, for example. You should be able to wear the looks you find. These particular stores tend to be on the trendy side and have quite a lot of clothes that you may like but that are not practical. If you don't like these stores, go to the ones you like and find the looks there.

Take a piece of paper and split it into two columns. On the left-hand side put a selection of your current formulas. It would be nice if you could take pictures of yourself wearing them (you don't need a lot of photos, just two or three of the ones that work the best, but you think they could do with being improved). On the right-hand side put a selection of the looks you want the most. Preferably, they should be the same formulas you wear. Then try to analyze the picture in detail (assess the color palette on the right and left sides, the overall mood, key items that are repeated, fabrics, prints or décor):

- Write down item-by-item, which clothes, strategies or tricks you already use in your wardrobe (it may be that you are already using the palette you like or certain accent items);
- Note where there are complete discrepancies (this is an important insight because this will be your primary goal in changing your wardrobe strategy);
- What, of the looks you saved, do you like in the abstract, realizing that it will probably not fit into your real life (for example, you might like it on someone else, but not how it looks on you) and what do you think will truly work for you in your day-to-day life? Think about every such detail: are you ready to try it out or look for compromises or should it just stay on your inspiration board;
- As the end result, try to make a list of strategies or specific items that you are ready to work on in your wardrobe (just write it straight out: expand my color palette, jeans should be looser, I need more fashionable bags, I should use multi-layering, and so on)

This exercise is for you to keep working on finding your own style and it will certainly raise your level of awareness of your stylistic needs.

I have a hunch that everyone knows about their silhouettes. Or is this the professional tunnel vision acting up? There are clear types, but life is stronger than any categorizing. You thought you were "nearly a triangle," but once you gave birth, you've got a strangely mixed-up figure...

The Theory of Body Types does work. It simply works with a single parameter – the volume at the top and at the bottom. We are well aware that there can be two women with the Inverted Triangle body type. One has a long neck, the other has a short one, one has a short torso and the other has a long one, one has a flat belly and the other does not. These are the nuances that the Theory of Body Types does not address.

If you are interested, here is a list of items for key body types. It's best if you look through this list with interest rather than awe, it is not the Criminal Code, after all. You may and should break the rules. If you're not interested, just skip to the next chapter.

INVERTED TRIANGLE

Is your body the inverted triangle shape? Then, we're looking for the list of the following items. Make sure you write this down, there's no fluff here.

In this case, the most interesting things happen at the bottom. For example, you have thrilling boots, then a small patch of bare skin, then amazing leggings, and you can cover up everything on top. You can use tops that flare out, tops with raglan sleeves, with a V or U neck or a halter neck.

You can go and Google Demi Moore; she demonstrates all this wonderfully. All her tops are monochrome and minimalistic with no ruffles, frills or decorations, whereas her jeans are stone-washed, ripped, or embroidered. You can wear flared or relaxed-fit pants, bright-colored or with prints. They should have a low waist. They can be baggy. Watch the movie Ghost. There, now for the skirts. They should have a low waist and be wraparound, trapeze or pleated; tulip skirts are also great. Jackets should go down to the hips and should be single-breasted; oversized ones work too. You should have A-line overcoats, straight single-breasted coats with a V neck, oversized or egg-shaped ones.

RUBENESQUE

Are you a Rubenesque woman? Then you need less decorations, ruffles, or pleats. You should not bustle and create an event; you are a beautiful event in your own right. You should not have to speak, but quietly place your sumptuous body above elegant shoes. Pumps with a square throat are a great option.

Loose tunics, wrap dresses, bottom-flaring shirt dresses are just right for you. You should wear plunging necklines and embroidered necks that remind us of times long gone. Wear flowing skirts, trapeze skirts, or straight ones. Loose knitted pants, evenly-colored jeans, pants with a low waist, and straight ones with wide legs all work for you. You have no need for all those holes, washed denim, or cargo pockets. On the other hand, an Empire line dress with a very high waist or a long dress with a plunging neckline would be just right. You can play at the 1920s, when the waist was worn low. Coats should be trapeze, A-line, or egg-shaped. There's no need to button your coat. Stylists say that this creates a vertical line, but all I see is Saskia, Rembrandt's wife, in the nude. There is so much love in that painting! Invest in accents and accessories. They'll suit you better than anyone else. Get rich purses and bracelets. Your story is all about luxury.

TRIANGLE

Is your body shape a triangle (they say, this is the most common type)? That means we focus at the top. You can use everything: hairstyle, earrings, scarves, puffed sleeves, tops with interesting collars or a round or square neckline, or even off-the-shoulder ones. The bottoms should be mid-waist or high-waist. Pants can be flared, palazzo, bootcut or straight. Wear midi skirts. Wear bomber jackets and straight or A-line coats. Egg-shaped coats are great too. This is not an exhaustive list, just the basic one.

HOURGLASS

We won't discuss the hourglass body shape. I think it's rather obvious.

Everything I am telling you here is based on classical principles of harmony. That's when we try to balance the top and bottom in triangle or inverted triangle body types or when we want to pinpoint a waist in a rectangle body type. In essence, we aim towards creating the hourglass silhouette. That's what pleases our eye the most. You can play with silhouettes and deliberately break up the usual proportions, but that is not what we are talking about here.

So if you have the hourglass body type, you would have to try very hard if you really wanted to ruin your natural silhouette.

RECTANGLE

Do you have a rectangle body shape? Then you should wear tops with voluminous sleeves or strapless ones. Wear halter necks. It is better to look at Gwyneth Paltrow many times than to read as many times about her. Wear tops with ruffles, decorated or with prints on the chest and shoulders. Wear T-shirts or blouses with deep, square or round necklines.

Generally, a woman with this type of body shape can create volume wherever she wants to attract attention. Bottoms should have a low waist, but there are a lot of exceptions. You can wear A-line skirts, as well as semi-circle or wraparound ones. Wear slouchy, bootcut, wide-legged, culotte, or flared pants. You can have pockets in your jeans that everyone else is banned from because they widen the hips. You should wear dresses with a plunging neckline or an open back, as well as high-waist dresses, A-line ones, kaftans, and kimonos. You can wear off-the-shoulder dresses. It is better to wear single-breasted jackets than double-breasted ones and wear

A-line, egg-shaped or oversized coats, as well as single-breasted straight ones and, bomber jackets.

Let's finish up with the dry official stuff.

APPLE

The apple-shaped body type. It is a little difficult to give universal advice here. Apple-shaped bodies are so varied; as are the other types. You should wear loose and straight tops and blouses with a V or U neck to enhance the portrait zone. You can also wear loose, long tunics and blouses or any tops with an asymmetrical hem and three-quarter-length sleeves. You can also wear trapeze, circle, semi-circle or wraparound skirts, and maybe even mini-skirts. It is better if your pants have a side fly. Wear dresses with a low waist in the 1920s style. You can also wear A-line, high-waist, asymmetrical hem, floor-length and plunging neck dresses, or shirt dresses. Your coats and jackets should be single-breasted, straight, or A-line or you can wear oversized and egg-shaped ones.

I know this chapter, like many closets, is full of doubles. But I simply must keep repeating myself. Find three or four formulas that work best for you and draw them in your notebook. Add up the doubles and extras. Assess how good the recurrences are.

Chapter Seven
Step #4 Meditative: Scale and Proportions

Do you wear clothes or do they wear you?

In the course of my forced experiment, a thought often crossed my mind, "I wonder if there is such a thing as custom-made jeans." There is a concept of an average person, but no such thing exists in real life. If it does exist, it is very, very rare and then, it is no average either. I am sorry for the triviality, but your clothes should fit you well. I am one of those who cut. I don't like to sew, I've no patience for it, but I have cut quite a number of things: neck tubes on sweaters, sleeves on T-shirts, and the length on skirts and pants, of course. Naturally, not all of my experiments were successful. And after every attempt at re-cutting something, I thought of becoming a self-designer and making my own clothes.

They say that the human mind prefers movement. The fifty-fifty ratio makes you feel stagnated. The eye prefers the two-thirds.

Sometimes, you think, "What a princess, I can't take my eyes off her. No, she's not a princess, she's a magician. A simple tee and shorts make a star!" Here's what the trick is: the length of the T-shirt is two lengths of her head, the shorts are one head-length. Add them together and you get 3.

According to the classics, the length of our body equals 8 times the length of our head. As a result, you get the 3:5 ratio (clothes – 3, body – 5).

The beginning of the Fibonacci series is 1:2, 2:3, 3:5. This sequence talks to us on a primeval level. It is used in architecture and in marketing. The Fibonacci series describes the position of rose petals. You come across it in music, in painting and in our everyday looks too.

Naturally, we are beautiful precisely because we are not perfect. Someone has amazingly long legs and a short torso, while someone else may have a long upper-body and short legs. Some have eight head-lengths in their body and some don't. What can you do?

Look for your beautiful lengths and find them. You already know them. The Fibonacci series is not just for roses, it's in our genes too. For example, the optimal length of a necklace is two head-lengths (your head plus one more). It is a beautiful balancing point.

This sequence works for volumes too. That's when something narrow and clinging at the bottom is compensated by double volume at the top or vice versa. When you dress that way, that's when your Fibonacci gene is most active.

So we look for magic helpers who know how to do alterations. You can't get away from them, because then your clothes would wear you, not the other way around.

These days, designers purposefully break the usual sequences or introduce them into clothes regardless of who wears them. You decide for yourself if you like this type of game.

Now, let's talk about the scale of things. What is the right scale? The print, the accessory, the buttons, the width of belts and lapels should be proportionate to your body. What is your scale as compared to the average person? Is your face large-featured or small? Have you had an experience when you tried on a coat and realized that it was all buttons and hardly any coat? Or have you come across earrings that looked like you borrowed them from Gulliver?

How about the scale of a stripe, for example? How does it talk to your facial features? If you're a lady of ample proportions, tiny thin stripes are probably not your thing. And vice versa, of course, wide stripes look clownish with delicate facial features. The same applies to the type of knit. Do your print, belt, or bag compete with your appearance for attention?

How can you look slimmer using a handbag? What do we do? We calibrate. We create. We produce hocus-pocus and illusions. Everyone knows about color harmony, but there is harmony in numbers too.

Fashion magazines and out-of-date books are full of this information. However, you can't use that knowledge because it has nothing to do with you. Your brain starts working when information is personalized. Unfortunately, I can't see you, so all I can offer is a few life hacks.

For example: the 1:1 ratio, despite its triteness. It often works because the outfit is in monochrome or because the wrists, ankles and collarbones are bare. Baring the thinnest and most elegant parts of the body is a technique that allows you to lighten the entire look. That is precisely why oversized looks so good in the summer.

The 1:2 rule and all the other commandments work better when you have a color contrast. It is the contrast that lets you see the separation. However, if you are wearing monochrome or shades that are close to each other, the rule doesn't work quite as well.

You can often see the shoe color chosen to continue the color of pants or skirt. This is the technique to make the rule of thirds work better; it elongates the silhouette because the color is the same from the waist down.

The general rule for choosing lengths (mini-skirts, boots, midi-skirts, and coats) boils down to the fact that you're looking for the thinnest and most elegant parts of your legs. You are not cutting them across the widest part, but are looking for a place where they begin to thin.

Chapter Eight
Step#5 Wardrobe Structure

Let's say that we can separate our life into four domains, just like our wardrobe: casual (home), business (work), semi-formal (the red carpet look), and romantic. You can have as many pieces in each domain as you like; it's all up to you. In the case of a capsule, we try to keep the number of items to a minimum. However, we need to solve the problems in each of these domains.

Why have I made these particular categories? You'll find the answer at the end of the book. In the meantime, I suggest that you accept this idea provisionally and review your wardrobe from this point of view.

Clothes are one of the tools you can use to achieve your life goals. If you are not happy with yourself in one of these domains, write down what is going on now and what you would like to happen. Dress for your future.

For example, your love life is not working out. Write down how you would like to see yourself. Just write three or four sentences or adjectives that describe you as you would like to be. You can even attach how you would like to look.

Remember how I talked about changing reality and about being the reason for and not the consequence of your circumstances? This is what this exercise is all about. In a sense, it is quite transformational. I can't promise you that it will work right away. Yet, many things will become clearer and you will understand what is going on in your life, in your closet and what direction you should move in. And that's half the job done!

Literally separate all your clothes into the four categories above. Make sure to include accessories (purses, shoes, jewelry).

So? Is it working? How many complete outfits do you have in each domain?

Obviously, the same items can be a part of different looks. Do you have, however, full and complete looks in all four domains? If you do and you like them, congratulations!

There are only four domains, but there may, of course, be forty four roles. Not every role requires a separate outfit. Uber Mom can also be a Good Neighbor and an Angry Housewife. A Banker can act as a Speaker, a Negotiator, a Strict Boss, or a Flirting Colleague. You can highlight the roles with make-up, for example, by painting your talking apparatus for the presentation or by including a bit of lace in the business image to denote the romantic side of things.

Do you remember my capsule experiment? Except for the casual domain, all others were just a glimmer, a hint. If I were happy with my capsule, it would have been one thing, but by February, Omicron, vitamin deficiency, and a move into a house with unfinished remodeling caught up with me. My heart yearned for love and celebration.

Would festive and romantic outfits have saved me? They may have done; they would have helped to reach out to beauty, to make the shift.

For now, let me leave you alone with your wardrobe. We'll meet again in the next chapter.

Chapter Nine
Step #6 The Basics

There is a concept of the so-called basic wardrobe. It is a set of items that play the part of workhorses. Non-basic items that play the role of accents go with them. I think everyone is familiar with this concept, which we are going to reconsider right now.

Let's try an easy test. Which of these sets would be included in the basic wardrobe and which wouldn't?

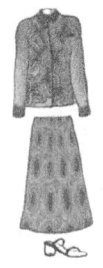

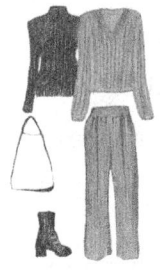

LET'S SHOP IN OUR OWN CLOSET

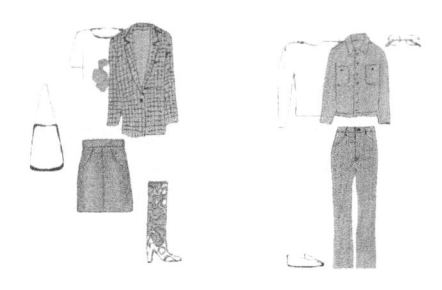

That's right! They are all basic.

What is basic? First and foremost, it is the CUT.

Many people think that we are talking about color and picture things in black and white or maybe in beige and blue. However, the basics don't mean a particular color; they mean the cut and the ability of every thing to work with each other thing. They can be of any color at all!

Let's take a simple shirt, for example. It is not just a piece of clothing; it's an epic piece of clothing. I suspect that when Dawnn Karen designed her famous convertible cardigan, she was inspired by shirts. You can roll up the sleeves, unbutton one or two buttons to show your collar bones or a necklace, or you can open it all the way, turning it into a cardigan of sorts. You can tuck it in or pull it out. You can use it as a first layer under a sweater or a top layer over multiple tops. And the color? Well, it can be any color; it all depends on the color scheme of your capsule.

Let me give you a list of clothes that are basic.

Please don't look at this list as 'what every woman should have in her wardrobe.' I personally don't have everything I've listed here. Look at it as a glossary or a reference list for what a basic wardrobe may include. It is huge.

So:

Footwear: riding boots, classic Keds, the simplest in sneakers, ballet flats, pumps, mules, sandals, loafers, ankle boots, and Chelsea boots. All of them are without bows, knots, several zippers, braids, draping, rhinestones, or other décor. Some metal is OK, like you see on most loafers. No weird forms of heels or soles. Every type of shoe is in its simplest shape and form.

Outerwear: a trench coat, a wrap coat, a straight single-breasted coat, a biker jacket, a denim jacket. Not fitted and, again, without decorations. Please understand me correctly: I am not saying that any other cut or design is not beautiful, I am defining what the basic wardrobe is.

Tops: a basic straight shirt, a T-shirt plus a long-sleeved tee, blouses: not fitted and with simple necklines (U,V, round or boatneck), without voluminous sleeves, interesting cuts or perforations, complicated darts, or open backs.

Trousers: Mid-rise or high-waist pants. Most pants are basic unless they have a lot of décor or are oddly cut. Straight jeans and pants, 7/8 length pants, mom's jeans, etc.

Skirts and dresses: linen dresses, straight dresses and skirts, A-line skirts from mini to midi without a lot of folds and not fluffy. Straight models are the base, we might have a bit of deviation; skirts might get narrower or wider. Dresses should be of simple cuts, without relief décor, interesting necklines or open backs; there should be no puff sleeves and they should not be fitted.

Jackets: full-length, simple, modern-cut jackets; they should not be fitted.

Bags: bags in simple geometric shapes (round, square, rectangular, trapezoid) without huge relief logos or other décor. City backpacks, not sports ones designed for hiking or other outdoor activities.

The list is not exhaustive. You can add to it based on your own sartorial experience.

I encourage you to choose basic modern styles, which does not mean trendy. Clothes must keep their structure and form, even if the style is casual. If a garment is associated with the following epithets: lethargic, flimsy, tired, sagging or shapeless, stop and think twice before buying it. The problem for many lies in the wrong size of clothes, as well as in wrong fabrics. No matter how well you work with proportions, flimsy, tight or shapeless fabrics only make the look worse.

Now let's talk a bit about modern fashion and global trends. After all, fashion responds with wardrobe solutions to everything that happens in society. What are good words to describe the strongest trend of the current decade? RELAXED. EGALITARIAN. ENVIRONMENTALLY AWARE.

What does 'Relaxed' consist of? It's the loose fit. It's not oversize; it's just that clothes fit you loosely in your comfort zone. It's an inclination towards natural colors and fabrics, the natural style in makeup and hair. Pronounced sexuality is no longer apparent in the looks; they are more intellectual now, as it were. The 'Egalitarian' in looks is reached by simplifying all of them. The luxurious is mixed with mass market and the pathos and drama are downplayed not just in sexual looks, but also in business and semi-formal. Nowadays, you mix tweeds with jeans, handfuls of pearls with chains and even different style clothes, such as a lingerie-style dress with sneakers.

In addition, Yin and Yang are fusing together. Lots of male clothes have moved into women's wardrobes and vice versa. If you wish to be in line with the times, but you like very feminine looks, instead of getting a very masculine jacket, get a silk shirt that's cut like a men's or work with a masculine print for very feminine clothes.

If we talk about 'Environmental Awareness' and conscious consumerism, we are talking about mini-wardrobes, the growing popularity of second-hand stores and re-sales, and new fabrics, such as eco-leather.

I would like to recommend considering the looks that stores like Farfetch offer. Not for buying anything there, nor for copying them thoughtlessly (their fashion awareness is often on the high side), but just to get in the spirit of the present-day and contemporary.

You have to agree that we can often decide on someone's age in a matter of seconds even if we see them far away. Age is betrayed not by wrinkles, but by outfits. A person dresses in the way they learned when they were young and then keeps that casing all life long. Is it important to be contemporary? Undoubtedly so.

Now, I would like you to assess how up-to-date your basic clothes are! It's an important step.

I cannot give you examples of all 'mothball' outfits and clothes. However, you can watch some movies that are ten or fifteen years old. Even outfits of the first seasons of such well-dressed TV series as *Suits* no longer transmit global trends.

I suggest that you compare your basics to similar items in online stores.

If your pants have pleated seams, but the seams are spreading along the thighs, it would make sense to replace them. It is the loose fit that will give you the feeling of slimness, comfort and fashion. Has it ever happened to you that you bought straight jeans but in reality they turned out to be a strange skinny hybrid? The fit was really tight even though officially they were called straight. That happened to me once. I looked at myself in the mirror and wondered how the so-called straight jeans managed to add so many pounds to my body. It is all about the interplay of proportions: straight jeans that fit even a little loosely make everyone look slimmer.

All of the above does not mean that I suggest you put half of your wardrobe in the trash. You can save quite a lot.

Tightly-fitting clothes, such as a cardigan or a denim jacket, for example, can be relegated to the bottom layer.

You can bring your look up to date by adding accessories. I don't wear glasses, but I can see how they can easily turn the mood of the look. Bags and shoes are excellent updaters.

Besides basic items there are challenging items, with their specific temperament due to too much texture or a complicated cut. For example, there may be ruffles sewed on to a top, or a leather jacket with straps, tags and studs, or complicated necklines. Such pieces are the divas that have a hard time cooperating with the rest of the team.

Let me give you a more common example: basic elastic-waist mom's jeans. If we were talking about light summer pants, I wouldn't say a word. Elastic-waist jeans, however, while comfortable, are not universal. That's because you will have to wear your T-shirt tucked in; and what if you want to wear it out?

Most people wear basic clothes. They are relatively simple and, most importantly, they can be in the most outrageous colors and prints. So the color comes to the fore. Let's make an experiment and make all eight sets in the picture above colorless. Now let's paint them any which way you like. As a result of this exercise, you have an incredible number of clothes.

Here is a pattern I've noticed. People either wear the basic cut and freely experiment with color, or they wear clothes of an interesting cut and texture but then there are restrictions on the colors or even simply monochrome clothes.

Now let us look at the basic wardrobe from the point of view of Will Hunting; that is – from the point of view of statistics and analysis.

What do people on planet Earth wear most often? What items of clothing does every person have? What is common for the rich and the poor, the programmer, the plumber, the top fashion model, and the future mom?

Jeans and jerseys! That's the actual basics, statistically proven.

Your basic wardrobe may be made up entirely of jeans-and-jerseys or you may have no denim in it at all, but in most cases, there's a mix.

All in all, I think you get the idea. Your capsule will be composed of basic items that work well with each other from the point of view of the cut.

Do you have a lot of non-basic items? Special ones with interesting texture or cut? What percent of your entire wardrobe do they make up?

Chapter Ten

Step#7 Color

Let us continue. How many color families live in your wardrobe? Do you have broken families, color orphans, mistresses, or even divas with a nasty temper?

I once read an article in the *Cosmopolitan* about an American writer. She had made a choice to wear only white. She believes that white looks snowy in winter and fresh in spring. She got married in a white tuxedo. This is just the case where you can step up to your closet and pick something to wear with your eyes closed – you'll never make a mistake. Her wardrobe is not dull. There are various textures: knitted sweaters, textured inserts, denim, leather, small insets of other colors in her sneakers. What does she get out of these monochrome options? Interplay of texture and no 'I've nothing to wear' pain.

I am not calling you to a single color, but to a single harmony. So, if you make up your mind to a capsule, color harmony is the key prerequisite.

What can I suggest as a quick and easy solution? Choose colors of the same saturation. Black frozen ground and red rowan berries give you one type of saturation; watercolors – another; ruby red wine and olives – a third. You can go the temperature route: warm and cold.

I already mentioned that all aesthetic instincts are intrinsic and that ninety percent of sane people who keep in touch with their bodies know everything they need to know about themselves. Colors are wave energy; it is physics. If you are obviously out of your color scheme, you feel it. Look at people in the stores, preferably people of different coloring: from a raven-head down to a platinum blond. You'll find that people simply don't see half of the products, they follow their call; they look for their own colors. This is basically what Johannes Itten wrote about.

I can just hear a question that's halfway a grievance, "What if everyone tells me that black is not my color, but I like it?" (Or something similar about other colors.)

Alright, you can wear it.

Wear it, but make it up in quality. Let it be a black evening dress, but an expensive one and well-made one. There must be energy coming from somewhere. If it's not in the color, then it should be in the craftsmanship or in the styling of the entire look.

When are we 'not in our color?'

When we dress for a part. When you're a professional actress, a model, an Instagram diva, or playing a part, no matter which one (we all do it fairly often). Like when you're the star of a corporate party, for instance. Or if you gravitate toward punk or rock styles: you have to agree that all fringes are partially role-playing.

Now, let's go back to where we started, to your closet. If we're going to talk about the capsule, it's best to give some thought to color. My experimental capsule had items that were white, anthracite-colored, and beige, shades of blue (saturated turquoise) and purple. Five-six colors may even be too much for some people. Remember that colors are reflected differently depending on the texture. For example, my jeans and bomber jacket were both blue, but they looked very different.

Write down, draw, or type up some draft ideas. What will be the basis of your capsule? What color scheme would you like to see it in? Select items according to how well they go together. I mean their color, cut and silhouette. Hang up the items that will be included in the capsule separately.

Chapter Eleven
Step#8 Capsule Wardrobe

You've already gone through your wardrobe in all kinds of ways. You've realized a lot of things about yourself. You have counted your clothes, looked at the colors, and reevaluated your formulas. You've got ideas.

Now, do you really think you need a mini-wardrobe construction set?

I should probably have put this chapter at the beginning of the book, but I really wanted you to read at least this far.

A capsule wardrobe promises you an incredible fairy tale. Even the word 'capsule' sounds like a magic pill. Just think about it: a wardrobe full of your favorite things that fit your lifestyle and where everything can be worn with everything else. The great advantage of a capsule wardrobe is that you buy less and you have more money for all the other fun things in life. The most important thing is that you feel beautiful and confident!

Capsule wardrobe is a modern trend. Many people think it applies to them. Let's think again before we succumb to mass hysteria.

How many changes do you need in your life? I am talking about everything. Do you have the same things for breakfast every day? Is your job creative or routine? Do you listen to the same music while you drive? What about your wardrobe?

You don't have time to think about how you look and prefer to express yourself creatively in your work? Or are you so fed up with your personal *Groundhog Day* that you'd love to give at least some variety to your daily routine through your appearance?

Are you ready to spend six months wearing twenty pieces of clothing? To get your drive from the same shirt (or pants) over and over again? As I said earlier, a minimalistic wardrobe (I mean the number of items) is just like a good basketball team where each player works with everyone else on the team. Each player must be the best in their domain and each one plays both the basic role and an accent one. That is why, unfortunately, clothes-divas or clothes that may be interesting to strangers don't belong there.

Since there are very few items, it is best that clothes be of good quality, up-to-date, and inspiring. You use and wash everything more often, so their potential is important.

Price. Would a mini capsule cost less? Most likely it would, but not always. The demands are greater; some of the things will wear out in one season and you'll have to replace them.

The advantages, on the other hand, are enormous. When you deal with a mini wardrobe, you save the energy on making everyday decisions. Your mind is not boggled by creating your look every day. When you open your closet, there is a lot of air and space and all the tops match all the bottoms, you can pick any set. You can be ready and buoyant in five minutes. You feel great because you've made a contribution to the prosperity of mother Earth. Then you can use the energy you've saved to read good books or do good works.

Let's discuss a different type of a wardrobe now. These are medium-sized or large ones.

You like to dress as the mood takes you, you are curious, and you like to try out new things. You like to experiment with texture, you like things to work as accents. You are even somewhat theatrical.

People with this type of wardrobe have a weakness, though. Imagine that you are putting together a book full of colorful pictures. In order to join all the pages together, you need glue and thread, that is – the basics. You go shopping and instead of buying dull glue and boring thread you buy yet another fun picture, that is – a self-sufficient diva. Your book never gets put together, but you like to look at the separate pages and ask yourself, "why is it I can never finish the book?" Sometimes, you take a grip on yourself and buy some glue, but it's cheap and of poor quality (why bother with expensive glue, no one sees it anyway) and so the book is glued together poorly. You may often see these wardrobes in the summer, where a collection may consist of up to 90% of fun clothes. Sometimes it is enough to buy a pair of white jeans and a basic T-shirt to glue some summer books together.

Price. If you have a medium-sized wardrobe, you wear clothes less often and they have a chance to last to the next season. Often, you can buy things on sale; I mean that if you have such a wardrobe, you can afford to wait for a sale. It is entirely possible that such investment will cost as much or as little as renewing a mini capsule.

Disadvantages. There is a great risk that your closet will turn into a mausoleum. Imagine that you have summer tops (tees, knitted and lace blouses, with a three-quarter sleeve or straps). Let's say you have thirty tops. You like them all. If you wear each top all through the summer, you'll wear each one three times. Naturally, they'll keep their look and, if you love them, will move on to the next season. Some of them will grow old: not mature like good brandy, but go sour like cheap wine. Even if you reduce their number, let's say you have fifteen instead of thirty, how many times will you wear each one? It comes to twice a month for each top. Then, there'll be a couple extras: a gift from mom, something you bought on vacation, and something so trendy that you couldn't possibly resist. That is how our closets become cluttered.

Quite a few people manage medium and large wardrobes very well. After all, the goal is not in the number of clothes but in being their mistress. However, any way you look at it, there is a capsule as the foundation of every well-managed medium or large wardrobe. There are several of them of varying dimensions. Sometimes, there are separate sets. There is no chaos in such a wardrobe or randomly accumulated items. You may be Spartan and live in twenty items for half a year, or you may have five capsules plus a couple of separate sets. If you can manage one capsule, you can manage five of them.

That is why, even if you think that you are the type for a larger wardrobe, you should still learn the principles of a capsule one. Start with the glue. Let there be several capsules of five to seven basic pieces in each. You can add interesting finds to them later on.

What about me? My closet is a yard and a half long. There is an area with shelves and another one with hangers. The top shelves house my situational wardrobe.

My wardrobe is not large, but it is not minimalistic either. I am still dealing with the aftermath of not-quite-strategic shopping. That is why I am now building mini capsules: by going shopping in my own closet. This is a strict and mandatory requirement. This is where you always start.

In my closet I find things that I rarely or never wore but that I like. Then the reactivation process begins: the drawing and planning. I must say, it's a lot of fun. Sometimes, it means a micro-investment: one inexpensive blouse that glues together several pieces. Sometimes, you hit a jackpot: a pair of summer shoes that are trendy and that were bought at a sale to boot. They can rejuvenate the whole summer collection.

Here is a piece of advice to those who are in the same situation as I am. Never shop without paying attention to your existing wardrobe. Start by finding good homes for the orphans, or hug them and give them to other parents. Start with them, with your ballast. You will often realize that in order to bring yet another piece to light, you'll need a fortune, not just a micro-investment. Even if it's not a fortune, you'll still end up with a small finicky capsule. Is it worth the investment? That's your choice.

There is one more rule: if you have acquired one item, another one needs to leave. You can get rid of two pieces instead of one.

Little by little, the chaos leaves. The blurred picture becomes clearer. Your wardrobe becomes more manageable. Is that not your true mission? To become the full mistress of your clothes and yourself!

Chapter Twelve

Step #9 On importance of Footwear and Bags

I'd like to talk about doubles and domains again, in other words, about categories of clothing.

For example, you have three skirts. They are different; they are not doubles either by cut or by color. But all three skirts are casual; they all belong to the same domain. However much you may try to create something semi-formal or business, it doesn't work. The same thing happens to accessories. For example, you bought two bags. One is square with a handle, over the shoulder and the other one is over the shoulder and rectangular. One is white, the other one is grey. You think that the white bag is semi-formal, possibly because of the color. But actually, both bags belong to the same casual domain. So it turns out that everything is in the casual domain and you keep asking yourself, "Why can't I create an interesting look?"

Every time before you buy a new accessory or a new piece of clothing, don't forget to ask yourself two questions. The first one is "Is this a double?" and the second one is, "To what category, what domain does it belong? What is the nature of this item?"

Some difficult readers might ask, "How do you determine which item belongs to which domain? It seems intuitively clear, but maybe it can be verbalized?"

It's a good question, but a literal answer may not take you to your goal. Let me explain.

Let's imagine three women.

The first one is elegant. She does not read fashion magazines but simply follows her esthetic instincts. When she works in her garden, it looks like Audrey Hepburn is having a photo shoot while planting flowers. She'd be wearing a shirt, a cashmere sweater and straight pants tucked into compound-colored rubber boots. She can't do it any other way. If she is going to a high-class event, she has no difficulties finding an outfit; she's in her element. To tell the truth, she finds it much harder to dress for gardening than for a glamorous occasion.

The second one likes things to be relaxed. She always wears jeans. If she's invited to a party, she wears jeans with a cropped tweed jacket and a handful of chains around her neck. She is smothered with compliments on her elegant look. She does look really cool, but strictly speaking, she is not wearing anything elegant.

Our third character is the veteran of the Boston Marathon. She loves sports and they love her. The most expensive things in her wardrobe are her running shoes and the gadgets that show how many minutes of REM sleep she had today. In a rare chink of free time, when she is not running, she goes to a non-alcohol party. She pulls on a knitted tee-dress, grabs a clutch purse and happily drinks in the compliments. Just exactly as if she were a First Lady. You must agree that it never really occurred to you that Michelle Obama often simply wears good-quality knitwear.

These examples show you that you don't have to understand yourself and your basic style, although it would be a very good idea. Whichever domain we talk about, it's actually all about you. You should not turn back on yourself and waste your money on something expensive to go out in that you will never wear. Some people look like a million bucks in a torn T-shirt and others need silks and velvet.

Personally, I promote the idea of an accessory base that changes the mood of the looks – see example below. I think that once we go through examples in this and the following chapters, many questions will fall away. If they don't, we'll have to meet on the pages of my future books where we'll talk about styles in details.

Real-life experience of a young woman

She wakes up in a good mood. That's because there's a regular day ahead, but she is ready for it! The lunch box for her son's school is bought. The shirt is ironed. And breakfast is just as delightful as the mistress of the day.

So, what's the plan? Take her son to school, then go grocery shopping, stop by the post office, and go to the bank.

Here goes.

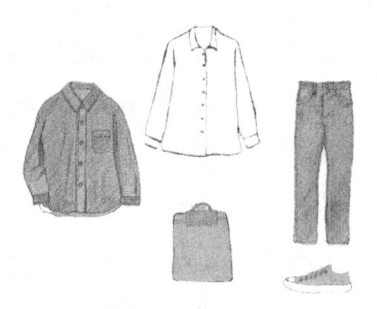

A nice adventure happened by the school. She saw Him again!

"With whom?"

"Alone with his daughter again. Why is he always alone? Where's his wife? Maybe he's divorced, just like I am?"

She walks her son to the school grounds as if accompanied by drums. That's her heart reacting to Him in a primeval rhythm. And the ripples up the spine…

"Calm down. Breathe slowly. Now, for the groceries and the post office."

She was walking dashingly to the post office along the line of parked cars, when one of the car doors opened and He stepped out. He was nervous as he addressed her.

"Excuse me, I often see you with your son and… I wanted to ask you, do you think you could go out with me today? This afternoon? Maybe we could have some coffee?"

The world stopped. She is just sitting there looking at the sky… How long has it been since she's seen Him? A half an hour, an hour? She is just fine sitting like that for the rest of her life. But the phone yelps, *Bank appointment*. Good Lord! The appointment is in fifteen minutes. Alright, time to run. Put up the hair, change the bag and sneakers. She can do her makeup at the bank.

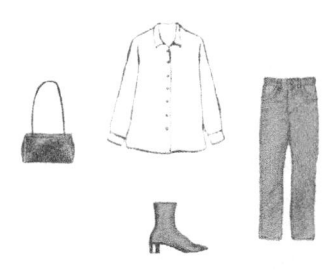

The line was still huge, even though she had an appointment. Any other time, she'd be annoyed, but not today. She got the loan too. Hurray! Got to run again. What if He hates waiting? She changes the bag and shoes again. She should take the scrunchie out of her hair. A bit of perfume… Well, here goes! She won't get any prettier.

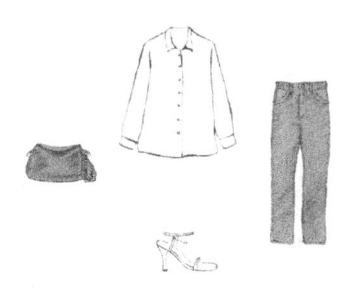

The date was great. But the day's not over yet. There is a long-awaited concert this evening. The babysitter holds the doorbell button forever. She runs to open the door with shining eyes. Here is her evening outfit.

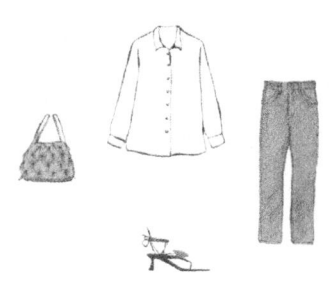

Let's not forget that a shirt is a transformer. If we're going to a business meeting, the shirt is buttoned all the way and is hanging loose. All the lines are crisp and focused. On the other hand, if we're going on a date, we can tuck it in half-way, unbutton a few buttons and pull the neck out to the shoulders or roll up the sleeves.

I think this is one of the most important examples. Of course, this is not a capsule.

Using a trivial set (a white shirt and jeans) as an example, I showed you all four domains (casual, semi-business, romantic, and semi-formal). See the role that accessories play; often, it is they that set the tone.

When you make up a look, you can start with a certain item. For example, you can take a dress and pick out accessories for it. But if you're a fan of basic clothes, it is accessories that help you create the right look.

Remember how we talked about global fashion trends and how pathos and drama are disappearing? The same kind of transformation is taking place in evening-wear. Actually, any routine look can be made into a semi-formal one these days. There is a very practical philosophy behind it: you're at work all day long and you go out at night. Going home where you can style your hair and change into something ornate is a waste of time and effort.

You need universal clothes for quick transformations. They may include midi skirts and pleated skirts, laconic mini skirts and dresses, culottes, jackets, shirts, any office outfit, lingerie-style clothes or satiny ones. If we talk about fabrics, then leather, denim, tweed, suit fabrics and satiny fabrics are very good transformers from a day-job to evening-out. Linen and knitwear, however, are much worse at it or they can't transform at all. All of the above clothes are basic.

What conclusion can we draw from this? Get yourself an accessory base that includes a pair of semi-formal shoes, a purse (anything small, not necessarily a clutch-purse), and a couple of fashion accessories and that's it.

I'll give you an example of such transformation further on.

Chapter Thirteen

Step#10 Business and Casual domain

Real-life experience of a young professional

Oh, no! Nothing good can possibly come out of this... The boss asked you to step into his office and shouted, "That's it! Your honeymoon's over. It's time to work on a real deal. You're going to N (a city with a branch office). You'll help them put together a leasing campaign. The project's been assigned to them ages ago and they keep dragging their feet. You're going to go there and work it all out."

You don't know anyone at that branch. Not only do you need to figure out what this leasing thing is, and figure out whom to approach with it, but you have to pack too.

No worries, I'll take care of the packing!

Day 1: You're going dressed for business, just like Terminator. You get off the plane and head straight for the office. There's a kickball game waiting for you, with you acting as the ball. That's why you need armor. Don't make it too easy to kick you.

LET'S SHOP IN OUR OWN CLOSET

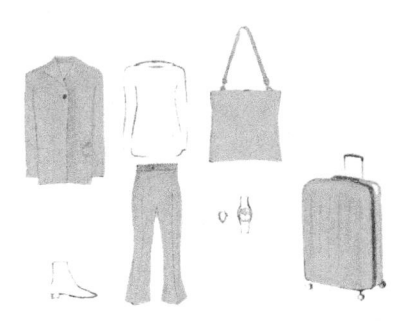

Day 2. You can take the armor off. The first day went like a charm. Apparently, you were expected. Maybe the management had some wicked thoughts about not taking you seriously, but as soon as they saw the rectangular silhouette in the door and a face camouflaging fear, they decided not to play with fire, or just to give you a chance.

The main stroke of luck on Day 3 was that there was a nice legal counsel who's just like you – just as smart and short on self-confidence. He's been assigned to head the project. Now you have certainly made a connection. He's invited you to a movie in the evening, so you don't have to spend it dismally on the hotel window sill. All in all, he needs people too. It looks like together you'll pull through with the project.

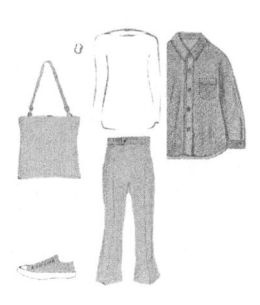

Whew! You've made it in three days!

I have already mentioned that a jacket is the present-day version of masculine armor. As soon as we start talking about anything official, we need a certain degree of a uniform or armor, its luster and smoothness of texture (remember medieval battle armor). Even high heels that make us look taller, are a type of attack, an additional weapon.

On the other hand, casual is when you lose form and drop your defenses, you've no one to fight. It lends itself well to flat-soled shoes. You've no need to announce over the loud-speaker that you work for such and such a company. Casual means creativity, informality, and unisex. These rules are not strict: the world changes and dress codes change with it. You can balance yin and yang. That's what I do, so as not to sink into sloppiness again. For instance, yang shoes are really good for joining together relaxed outfits, whereas sneakers relax business suits.

Chapter Fourteen
Step#11 Building capsule

Example#1

Imagine a woman who is a Kate Winslet's type (color type), an average woman with two small children (a five-year-old and a three-year-old). She only shops for clothes when mass market retailers offer sales. Nearly all the clothes in the examples come from these stores.

She has good taste (who doesn't?). She shops chaotically because she has no time or energy to spare. She has not cleaned out her closet in a couple of years. She's got everything but the kitchen sink in there.

She was going by a huge shop window, when she saw this. She was amazed.

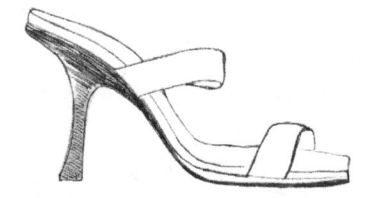

Expensive? Oh, yes! But that's not the point. It suddenly dawned on her that it was spring. For so many years, spring just flew by, with the kids being sick, with sleepless nights...

It was time. Time to think of herself. She bought them. With her heart thrumming, she asked herself, "What is it that I just did?" She spent nearly her annual budget on clothes.

But she didn't have the heart to take them back. Instead, drunk with too much sun and the song of a starling, she ran home. To heck with cleaning, cooking, and everything else! Today, the day is just for her. She had just one goal in mind.

She knew just what to do. So, where was that book? What book? The one about shopping in your own closet. It'll come together. Her subconscious knew what that closet was full of.

All the windows were open. Kids were playing outside. There was a pile of clothes on the bed.

She'd take a few basic items and it will all work out. She knows her formulas and what suits her. She just needs to deal with the chaos in the closet.

So, the beige suit has never let her down. Then three tops: the first top is a sleeveless blouse, but not the one with thin straps, the second top is a T-shirt with a print, the third is a basic beige tee. Then, there is the wine-colored sweatshirt, the white shirt, the pink cardigan and the flowing skirt. How many items does that make? Nine. Now for the shoes, she'll have three pairs: the ones she bought today, loafers, and sneakers. How about accessories? That would be one or two scarves, a belt, three bags, a baseball cap, and a chain.

Remember the example with jeans and a white shirt? The logic here is the same, a very simple one. I am sure you've noticed that there are only two bottoms in the capsule: a pair of pants and a skirt. Our character will make sets out of the basic items she chose. She'll play with accessories adding character to her looks. Remember, she needs complete looks for casual and business situations, as well as something for romantic and semi-formal ones.

What has she got for the tops? There are three second layers: a jacket, a cardigan and a sweatshirt and four tops: a sleeveless blouse, two T-shirts and a shirt (the shirt will work as a second layer too).

Let's look carefully at each of the items she picked.

Please, I know that my drawings are not super.

PANTS

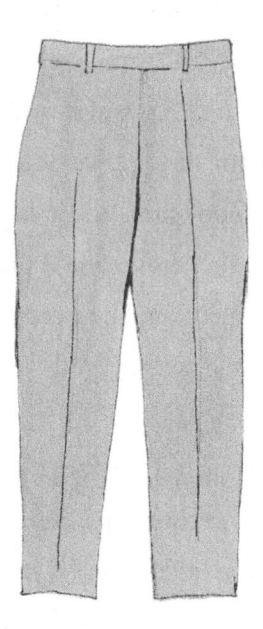

I would recommend such shortened pants to practically everyone. Everybody would have their own type, of course. The pants should not fit too closely, especially the part below the knee. If they are light summer ones, then they often stop above the ankle bone and work marvelously with high heels. Overall, the perfect length for such pants is to the ankle bone. You can also have them in a heavier fabric, such as suit fabric, for example, and then use flat-heeled shoes: loafers, sneakers, or wide-heeled boots. Our character decided to hit two birds with one stone: she chose light-colored suit fabric. You can wear anything with such pants: from sneakers to heels.

SKIRT

It's the universal A-line. It is flowing and above the ankle. Despite the fact that it is not made of heavy thick fabric, it can easily migrate from summer to fall and winter. Such a skirt can be pleated or wraparound.

LET'S SHOP IN OUR OWN CLOSET 69

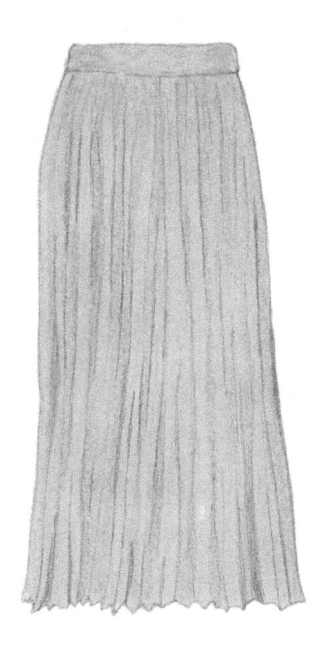

SWEATSHIRT

She chose the sweatshirt because it is smooth and holds the shape better than many pullovers or jumpers. The texture also works better for women of the Kate Winslet type.

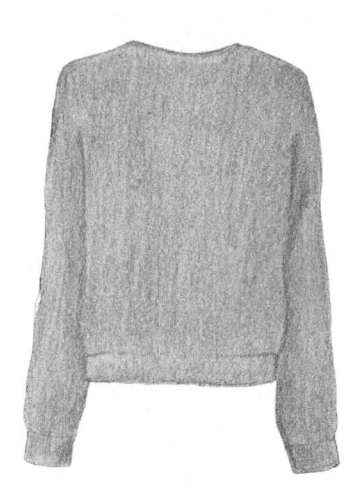

Now, I am going to digress and talk about style a little. If we start with appearances (which is not quite right, of course), you want to dress a woman of the Kate Winslet type in the elegant style, even if you are going for athletic looks. The keys to the elegant style are a smooth, soft fabric (if it's knitted, cashmere works best), absence of sharp lines, high necklines, monochrome or smooth shading look good, no decorations, such as patch pockets or accessories, shawls and scarves without fringes. Summer women and some Winters dress that way. We'll talk about them in the second part of the book.

SHIRT

We already talked about the shirt. Let me remind you of our meditative step on scale and proportion. If your facial features are large and the collar is narrow, the head will appear even larger and the features larger yet. On the other hand, if you have delicate facial features, you might sink in a large collar.

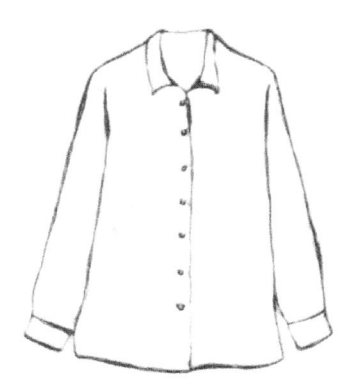

CARDIGAN

I don't want you to think that everything is simple and easy. It is very difficult to pick a good cardigan. There are a lot of these shapeless things. It is best not to be carried away by them and their sisters – voluminous sweaters with a high neck. You can sink into them up to your ears. As soon as you feel that you are blurring, give yourself shape and form. It is best to pick cardigans without pockets, so that nothing stretches and make sure it is of high-quality, close knit.

A mix of textures makes the looks interesting. For instance, a light floating silk dress, in this case with a light skirt, would look beautiful with a knitted cardigan. You can emphasize the waist with a medium-sized belt about an inch or inch and a half wide.

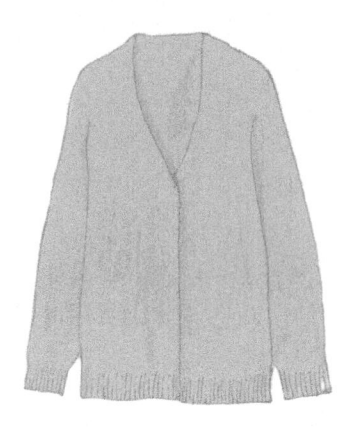

TOPS

Tops are the part of an outfit that manages the mood. You can make a ton of combinations with a single pair of pants. Tops, especially T-shirts, are not particularly expensive, but that is the whole problem. You can replace tops more often, but please, don't get carried away. Think about how much money you spent on several tops and what piece of clothing or accessory you could have bought instead.

The tops that our character chose fit her loosely. They are not oversized, but there is air between the body and the fabric.

The first top is a blouse in smooth, satiny fabric. It's leaning towards the elegant, but it is, nonetheless, universal. You can wear it either with Bermuda shorts or with office trousers. It can complement all looks: casual, romantic, business, and semi-formal. The wider straps are more universal, so is the V-neck.

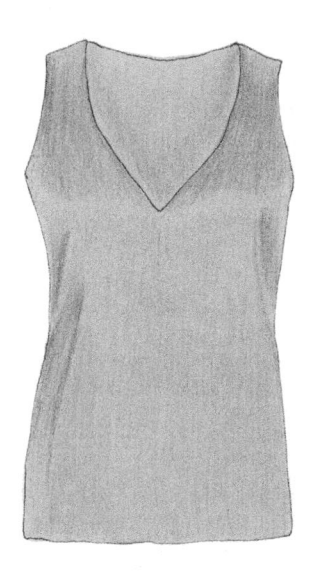

There is a semi-close-fitting tee with a print and a solid beige one. As strange as it may seem, T-shirts are also universal. They lean towards casual, but it does not mean that you can only wear them with shorts in the summer. They can fit business looks very nicely with office pants and accessories. If your dress code is not too strict, you can wear them to work. The important thing is that they should be of high quality and have an interesting print.

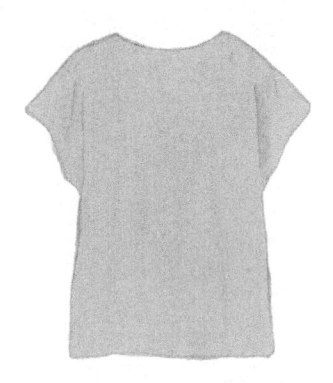

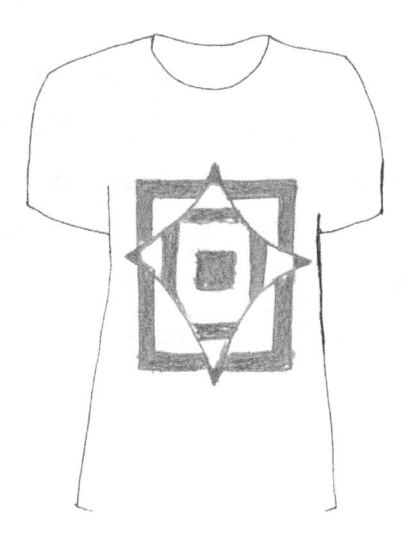

JACKET

This is not the simplest of categories either. I already mentioned that this is the present-day version of medieval armor. So everything is important in this complex structure: the shoulders, the length of sleeves, the lapels (are the lapel lines soaring up or are they pulling down, or maybe you don't need lapels at all), buttons (what color are they, are they decorative, do they pull you down, how does their size work with the scale of your face), pockets (do they make the look heavy), fabric, and color. If you shop online, make sure to check out the model's height and how it looks on her. If your height is less than 5'6", it is best if the length of the back is around 25 inches. If you are taller than 5'6", it can be around 30 inches. Our character chose a straight jacket that is not baggy.

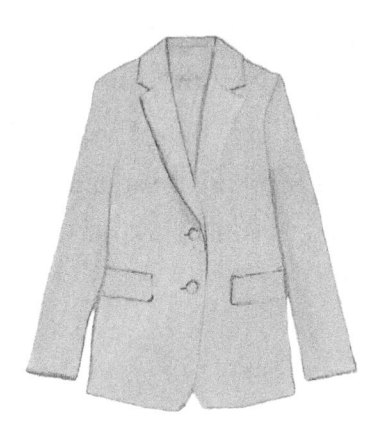

SHOES

There are three pairs of them in the capsule and they are all different types. Together with the rest of the team, they create either more relaxed or more formal outfits.

Now, let's see the looks that can be made here. They consist of a series of outfits with pants and skirt.

I think it's time to discuss accessories. They are to a look, what spices are to a dish.

If you don't add salt, your dish will be bland. If you forget to add pepper, it won't be hot. If we don't put in spices or herbs, we may never find out what the dish tastes like at all. The Chinese note five flavors: hot, bitter, sour, salty, and sweet. We have to have each of them every day. So should our looks be completed, combining things that seem incompatible at first glance. They should include no less than five items. Count how many pieces of clothing you are wearing, including accessories. If you are wearing less than five, there is a risk that your look is not complete. Look at yourself in the mirror. Is it bland or have you overdone the spices?

What do you do with accessories? You need to try to wear them. It is not easy. I am not really a guru in the field. I look at headwear and realize that a hat can take the most hopeless look to a new level. I still don't wear them. I'm always happy to buy another pair of shoes, but I simply don't see hats. A baseball cap is the only thing I accept without a struggle. But that's alright, I am sure I'll grow into them some day.

I won't talk about all the possible accessories, but only about the ones used in the capsule.

BAG

We have three of them.

There is the one and only. It's not too large, about the size of a small book. The scale is important here, pick the one that works for you. In any case, it will not be a large bag that you can put your laptop and groceries in. It ought to give your look lightness. I recommend that you pick the one that works for all seasons. If it's not too dark it will look light in winter against darker clothing and it won't be too heavy-looking in the summer.

The key criterion of basic bags is that they should be of a simple cut (oblong, square, trapeze, circle, or triangle), although they may have rounded corners. But the most important thing is that they should hold their shape. They should not be baggy, or shapeless, or tired-looking, like a dumpling left in the sun. They should be *al dente*. Even if you buy a dumpling-bag, it should still be *al dente*! I can't explain it any other way. The rigidity and energy of shape will save the flowing summer looks and will add spice to any casual look. Also, they need to be up-to-date.

The choice of a bag is tied closely to the color palette of your capsule. If your capsule is monochrome, the bag can have a print of the key capsule colors. If you don't like bright accents, then you can have a monochrome bag with an interesting texture: quilted, embossed or textile.

I must turn your attention to a set of separate accessories closely tied to bags. They are bag belts and handles. You may have several. For example, you may have a beige bag with a simple beige belt, with a chain, and with a printed belt.

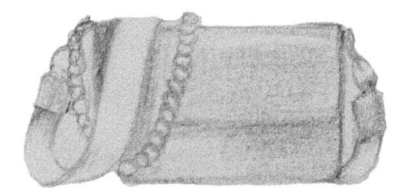

Second bag. It is more functional; you can fit half your life into it. All the comments on the first bag also apply to the larger one. The size and level of relaxation of the bag depend on what you need it for. Do you need it for your laptop and paperwork, for groceries or for baby things? The bag in the capsule is relaxed and more athletic.

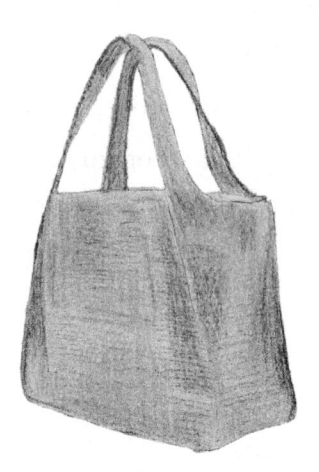

The third one is something small.

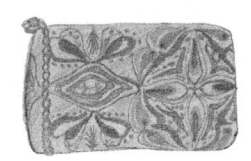

BELT

It is not necessarily an accessory. However, if you wish to emphasize your waistline, why not give your outfits a good belt? You can wear belts with jeans, trousers, dresses, over cardigans, jackets and outerwear. A belt gives you a color accent and pulls the look together.

They are especially good for multi-layered looks. A belt may echo the bag or the shoes, but it doesn't have to. Overall, a belt, better shoes (in other words, non-athletic ones) and a rigidly-shaped bag are very good for pulling together sloppy casual looks.

Let's define the difference between a waistline and a belt. The key difference and advantage of a belt is that it provides you with a different texture. It is this difference that makes the look interesting, even if you're wearing monochrome.

Start with a simple belt for jeans, about an inch and a half wide, with a regular buckle. It is best if you can tie it in a knot. In that case, you'll be able to use the belt with all your clothes. Once you make friends with a belt like that, you can go to belts that are wider and more interesting, with a pretty buckle that would chime in with other accessories.

A wide belt is around 2 inches. Don't forget about scale and proportion. You have to calibrate. It may very well be that an inch and a half is your preferred width.

A PENDANT OR CHAIN

Pick the kind that goes well with both a knitted tee and a sweater. Just as with the belt, it's a story about the contrast of textures. Besides, this type of accessory always brings an outfit to life. You need to bear in mind the same balance here – whether you pick a chain or a pendant, they have to be visible, but not obtrusive. If a chain is not very visible but you love it, wear it by all means. In that case, I suggest that you add something larger and more noticeable to it.

SCARF

A scarf is like a cherry on a cake. If you make friends with this type of accessory, you can transform and beautify the most trivial outfits. However! A cake that has gone sour or was burnt cannot be saved by a fresh pretty cherry. So, no scarf can possibly save a nondescript, bungled look.

1 SEMI-FORMAL

ALAYA AIFEL

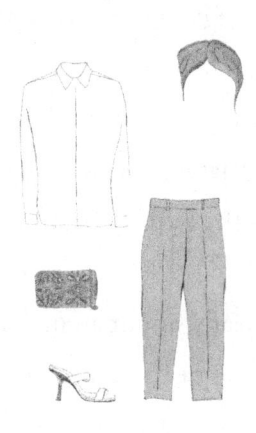

2 FORMAL

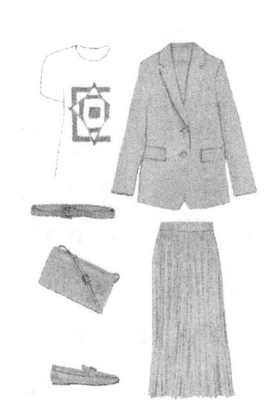

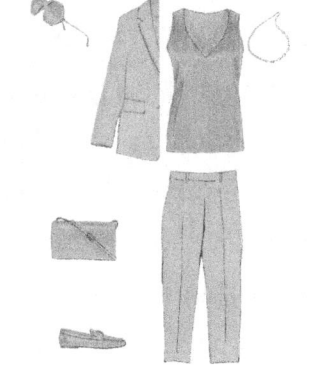

3 CASUAL

LET'S SHOP IN OUR OWN CLOSET   81

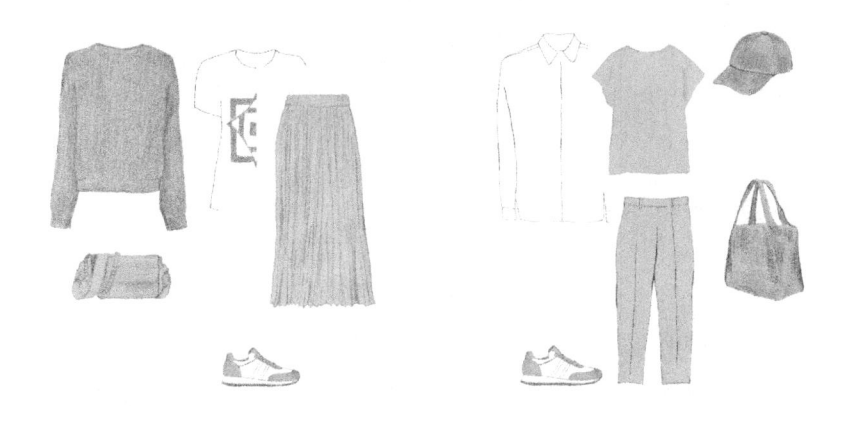

4 ROMANTIC

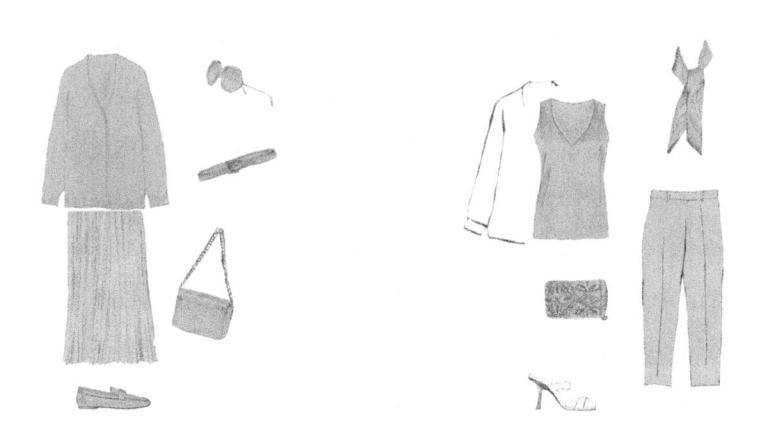

Some would think that the capsule is boring. I might agree. It is very neutral and could be edgy.

Some may think that this is a lot of work and you'd be right. But it's worth it. You can make the capsule even more interesting by adding style-forming items. However, I wanted to show you that the simple basic clothes are enough.

Overall, this capsule is a bit about present-day femininity. It is a neutral base. You can go deeper and make it more personal. You can go into elegance, sports, or relaxed fit.

Example #2

Let's try again.

If anyone asks me, "What criteria of appearance are the most important and at the same time the easiest to understand, so they can be used as a springboard for building a wardrobe?" I would say that it's the contrast of appearance.

What I mean here is the contrast between the color of hair, eyes, and skin. I think that understanding your personal contrast is easy. The easiest way to determine it (if you're still in doubt) is to switch a photo of yourself to black and white. Your contrast level may vary from low to high.

This criterion gives rise to two ways of creating a look. Both of them are good and work for all types, regardless of contrast level. However, I noticed that people with less contrasting appearance tend to use the second method, whereas people with high contrast use both equally successfully.

The accent method. Very bright and sometimes even exotic items are used to create a look. For the purposes of this book, we use 'accent' as it relates to color or texture, not the cut. A large item, such as a skirt, a jacket, a coat, or a dress can work as an accent and the look is built around it. Some women with a soft, low-contrast appearance (but not all, by any means) may be lost behind such a vivid piece.

The other method, as you probably already realize, is the opposite of accent. The previous capsule was made for a character of Kate Winslet type, where the contrast level was not very high. Everything was soft, practically all the colors were of the same saturation and there was no great contrast between them. The looks were often created with analogous colors, similar in shades; for example: blue – blue spruce – green. There is complete harmony among all the details of the look. Bright colors were used only as a sprinkling to invigorate the look and overall, such looks are more reserved, elegant, and dignified. When you use this method, the shades and textures of clothes come to the forefront.

Now, I suggest we build a capsule for a brunette with a fairly high contrast level. We'll use the accent method.

Actually, the capsule you see below is even reserved for this type of appearance. You can make it even more striking or totally insane by adding accent accessories or printed items. As long as our character likes it, this riot of colors looks very natural.

There is a streak of masculinity in the capsule and we have built looks in all four domains

Let's call the color scheme for the capsule the Vitamin Queen.

It should appeal to your primordial instincts and use old, ancient colors. Many centuries ago people used to recognize only three basic colors: black, white, and red.

You can read about it in the stories: "A witch in black robes gives a red apple (which is poisoned…) to a young girl whose skin is white as snow." "A black… [crow] drops a piece of white cheese, which is grabbed by a red fox." "A little girl dressed in red carries a pot of white butter to a grandmother (or a wolf) dressed in black." The color triad (white, black, and red) was one of oldest. "…Chess… throughout its history has opposed either a black side to a red side, red to white, or white to black." "There was no place for blue, yellow or green in this three-color system."

Now let's construct the capsule. I think it was Coco Chanel who said that all a woman needs is a couple of suits and one dress. We will use that great legacy literally. We'll put together two 'suits' and pick a dress. The brightest accent is the tee. Everything else is quite reserved, but it is for a high-contrast type of appearance.

I built this capsule for three domains: casual, business, and romantic. Try to step back from the particulars and look at it as you would at a diagram.

My sets are pant suits. If you don't like pants, you can put together skirt suits. Try to play a Sudoku of sorts, combining the items with each and every one. They have to be compatible with each other.

I'd like to bring your attention to the fabrics; they are very important. For example, if your white shirt is a little softer or more transparent, it would no longer have the business look. A softer and more transparent shirt may be several times more expensive, it may have exciting decorations, but no, it won't work.

So, we look at fabrics. (Here, you can picture me nagging you on the subject for the next fifteen minutes. It is quite boring, so I would just ask you to embrace the idea.)

You can have twice as many tops. That way, you'll have seven pieces of clothing and two pairs of shoes. It would be best if the tops you add to the family are not doubles. That way you will have seven unique items in your capsule. All in all, you can live in seven items. Here, the question is how often you do laundry and how fast does it dry.

LET'S SHOP IN OUR OWN CLOSET

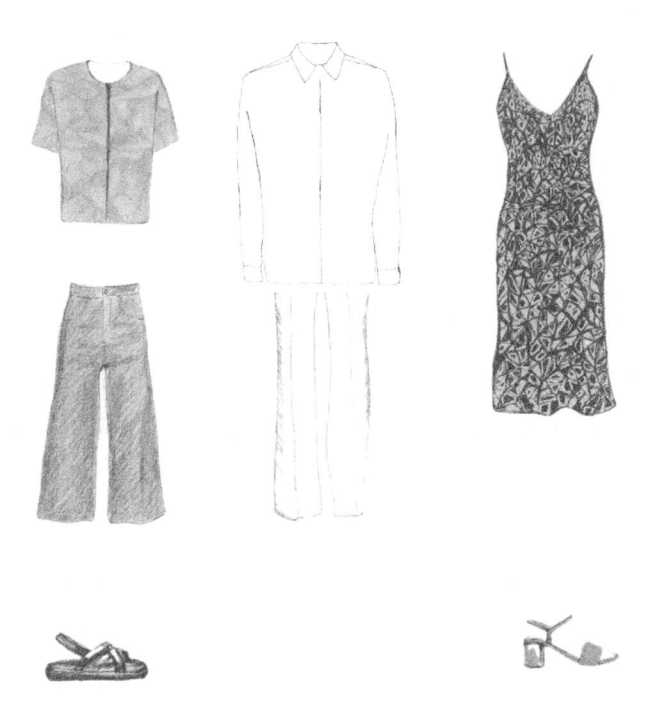

Let me emphasize the key idea of the capsule wardrobe one more time. You don't want doubles (either color or silhouette ones). A capsule is a team of unique pieces of clothing. For starters, try to put together a capsule of five items.

I've talked about color a lot already. Turn off the colors that are there and paint your capsule whichever way you like. You can have wild combinations: a print over print or screaming neon colors. Alternatively, you can go for quiet, muted colors.

If your life is more in the casual domain, we can add one more "suit". If you want more dresses, expand that domain. Are you a business woman? Then we'll add to the business collection.

The capsule is missing accessories. I would add a couple of bags (a backpack and a small purse), a shawl and hair accessories. That's what it looks like in my imagination. You can dress it any way you like.

If the weather is cool, let's add a trench coat and a sweater.

Example#3

This is the last example. Let's build a capsule for a medium-contrast appearance. Let it be a brown-eyed, chestnut-haired lady who works from home and likes natural, easy looks. Relaxed is her middle name.

People with medium-contrast appearance can wear softened contrasts. So they can have a black and beige, for example, instead of black and snow-white. They have a huge range of color combinations, except the most extreme ones.

We'll build a mini capsule with the same basic clothes.

How do you get relaxed? That's easy. You let go of geometry and strict forms. You take on soft shoulders and skip the accents either around the waist or at any other part of the body. Use cotton, denim, linen, soft leather or suede and, of course, knitwear. Everything is as comfortable as possible. Use everything that looks natural and a bit used, such as tarnished silver or scuffed jeans. As a rule, people who like this style don't use very bright colors or prints. On the other hand, there is a lot of multi-layering and texture variance.

If our first example was a bit on the feminine side and the second leaned towards Yang or masculinity, this third example is more about unisex.

Just as in the previous examples, you can start with these sets and go to pertness, pastoral romanticism or mix the relaxed with the minimalistic.

LET'S SHOP IN OUR OWN CLOSET

Please, be indulgent towards my drawings. Imagine that the brown shirt, regardless of its formal appearance, is made of flannel or wool. The skirt is eco-leather. The color palette is from milky-white to brown.

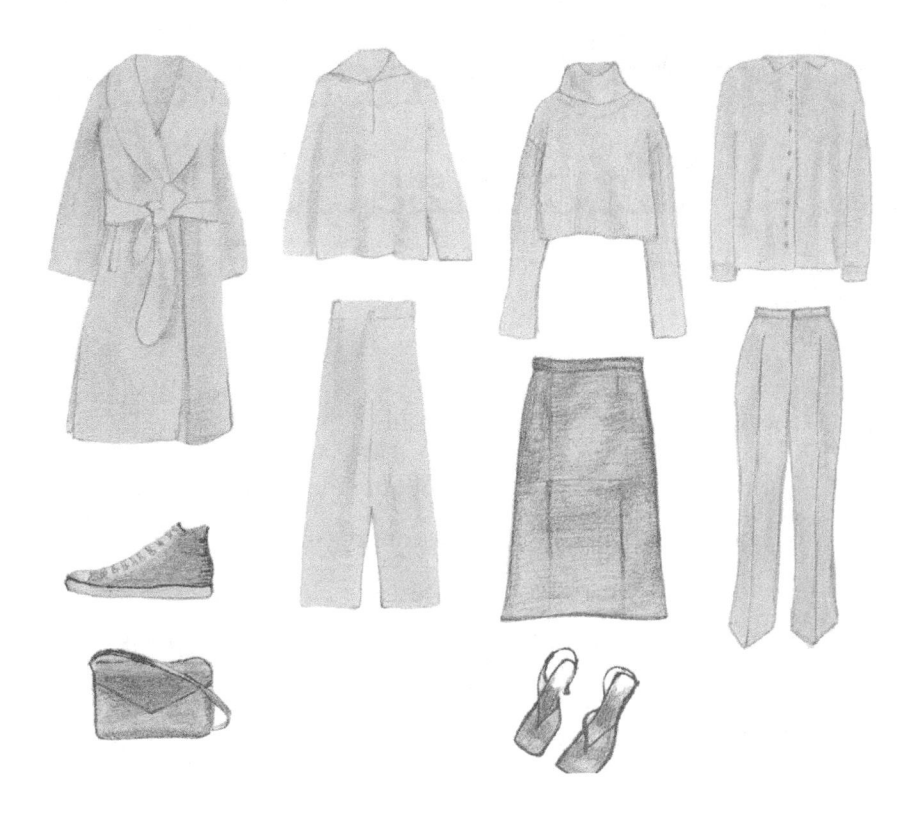

Chapter Fifteen
Step #12 Concept and Vizualization

How do we move towards our capsule?

Just as if we were in a jungle. We use the suggestions in the book as we would a machete, clearing the way towards our dream. We've a vague notion in our minds, elusive as a mirage.

I am a hundred percent certain that for some of you the paths are still overgrown and not well cleared. But they are there! They've been mapped out. And the most important thing, of course, is that you are on your way.

Here's a question for you.

Do you have a concept?

"What's that? We haven't talked about it. Please, just let me deal with the chaos in my closet!"

Right now, you are most likely going towards your capsule without a concept in mind. That is just fine, that's what most people do. That's what I did too, straying and making a huge number of mistakes.

For many people, simply working out the "up-to-dateness" of everything is a huge step, for others, picking five to nine items and stepping into the capsule world is just like conquering Mount Everest.

But then, there are others. There are those for whom such goals as "everything matches everything else by color," "fewer clothes that all work with each other," and "everything is up-to-date" are a matter of course, they are not even goals. They need more.

In the first case, the suggested algorithm works just fine: you think through the capsule palette, pick out the models that suit your body and textures, pick out the minimal wardrobe of basic clothes, then introduce accessories that match the palette and are neutral.

In the second case (when you build your concept), it all boils down to your own style. The algorithm is not very different from the first case. All you do is add the spice of the proverbial *your own style* to it.

You go back to the very beginning. Study your notes and your favorite clothes. We have already done the exercise I am suggesting here. Find the four looks you want: I am semi-formal, I am romantic, I am business-like, and I am casual. Try to formulate the concept in just a few words. It would be great if you can come up with fun names. Something like, Fun Homeless Housewife or The Office Feminine.

Then, you pick a few key items and accessories that would reflect this particular spice of yours and introduce them to the capsule. This is not easy. If you are not quite clear about what you want your wardrobe to do or if you want too much, don't make it too complicated, just keep going as you are, without a concept. It'll be right there, waiting for you once you clear the chaos in your closet.

Whichever option you chose, it won't happen without a fair amount of planning and in any case you will have, if not a fundamental concept, then at least a fair idea.

I am not a great fan of visualization, I am more about trust.

BUT!

There are areas, quite a lot of them, where it is absolutely a must. Such as building a capsule wardrobe, for example.

Imagine that you need a new kitchen. What happens? You go to a professional, who draws your new life for you. The color, décor, and functionality of the kitchen are very carefully chosen. Everything has a bearing on your decision: the price, the quality of materials, as well as your taste. The process may take several hours or even days and you then have a visual idea of what it will be like in real life.

Does your wardrobe deserve less attention than your kitchen? You can argue, of course, that buying a new kitchen is a large investment! Have you ever added up all the money you've wasted on clothing and how much unhappiness you've experienced by being shorted on the joy you deserve to have?

I suggest that you get together the photos of things from your closet that will take part in your capsule, as well as photos of things you potentially want to buy that you took notes on.

The important thing here is to create a visual presentation. You don't have to buy that particular Burberry coat. You are looking for the whole picture. Later on you can find something similar in your price range.

Don't torture yourself by digitizing all the looks and new acquisitions. Although... why not? Imagine that you need to put together an evening outfit quickly and solve a bunch of problems at the same time. A photo will show you what you should wear at a glance. I don't know whether you would have the time to digitize everything, though. However, I am positive that a single glance at a capsule that shows you the entire color palette, the cut and nature of the clothes will help you move towards building your wardrobe tremendously.

Remember we talked about a smart wardrobe? It means smart and efficient shopping. Plan and plan again! Stop being a hostage to circumstances.

A picture you can see also helps you to plan if you cannot afford to buy all you need at once. In addition, it helps you not to be distracted by emotional shopping.

Don't skip this step!

Chapter Sixteen
Step#13 Summing up

Now, I will try to systematize everything I told you about and add to it.

As you must realize, I used the one-capsule-for-four-domains method. I haven't even touched upon such a domain as sports, which makes up a huge chunk of life for some people, nor the summer-capsule-for-travel, nor the at-home capsule, nor a number of other situations. What you do, for each such situations is you build a micro-capsule. Naturally, clothes from the main capsule can be used for any of the others.

You can go the multi-capsule way. That's when you come up with a capsule for each of the four domains plus micro-capsules for a few other limited situations. In this book, however, I did not focus on the multi-capsule approach.

How do you build a capsule? It is best to start in the season you are in right now.

The single-capsule method presumes that there are universal players. All in all, the smaller the capsule, the more neutral and universal should the clothes in it be.

Technically speaking, you start building the capsule with outdoor clothes and end with accessories. Life, however, overpowers any method – our closets are overflowing, yet there is nothing to wear. That is why we

LET'S SHOP IN OUR OWN CLOSET

used the method of clearing the wardrobe and finding the framework, in other words: working formulas made up of your favorite clothes. All we need to do after clearing the ballast is to put the puzzle together, to find the missing KEY pieces of clothing.

Let's say you found one powerful outfit, build on it. Separate it and start building other outfits, adding new pieces and keeping in mind what domains you are building them for. To fill in the gaps, make a list of the key pieces you need. As soon as you manage to put together outfits for all four domains, your capsule is done. Finish up with the same accessories, because a bag, for example, is a binding, linking element and we want it to match everything.

Start with the bottoms! Think of two bottoms that would work in all situations. They may be a pair of jeans and a skirt. On the other hand, are jeans truly universal? If your dress code at work allows it, they may work. If you start with a universal minimum, you can take it all the way down to one pair of formal trousers and a skirt. They work for everything.

Let there be trousers. They will be your pants that fit you personally by cut, fabric, and color. Now you need to pick the first layer and the second, shoes, outerwear, and accessories. Try to put together four functionally different looks based on one pair of trousers. Now add another bottom that is not a double. Let it be jeans. Put together four outfits and add the tops. Keep in mind your color palette and compatibility of clothes.

Imagine that you have a startup. Let it be the startup of a school. Your bottoms are the first tier of management: the skirt is the school principle, the pants are the head of teaching, the jeans are head of operations. They have to hire their team. Every new colleague has an interview with every boss and a mutually enriching dialog should take place with every boss. In other words, you start with the bottoms and have every top go through each bottom. Some tops go with everything – they would be your startup candidates.

What about doubles and extras? Yes, you can have a few extras, but only talented ones. Don't overdo them or you'll be drowning in an overflowing closet again before you can say *style*.

Anything else you add is optional, but it's a good idea to have it. It may be a one-piece, such as a dress or a jumpsuit, or it may be a skirt.

Now, let's look at your capsule from another point of view. What does it consist of?

It's made up of basic clothes, but they can also be separated into neutral pieces and accents. Accents, for example, may have a different texture or color or a print. Trendy or fashionable basic items can also be used as accents. For example, you can have shorts, but make them leather, a super-trendy pair of shoes (that are still universal), or a sleeveless tee of a trendy cut. If the backbone of your capsule may last many years, there is a risk that the trendy basics will have a much shorter lifetime, it all depends on how practical and robust the particular trend is.

There are several stylistic tricks you can use to make your basic wardrobe exciting. They are multi-layering, playing with colors and prints, and introduction of different textures. Let's take the different textures, for example. You are wearing seemingly simple clothes, but people can't take their eyes off you and want to keep looking you over and over. That's because you are wearing matte leather trousers, a knit jumper of a similar shade, a bag with an interesting finish and shoes that echo the bag. Everything is extremely simple; they are basic clothes in quiet colors, but the look is complete and interesting.

And now, let's have a list again.

Actually, it's right there in "The Basics" chapter and many pieces have been demonstrated in the capsules, but I have a feeling that we could use the same thing expressed a bit differently.

Please, do not read the list as "you must have it". Remember, we started with the most viable combinations that work for YOU.

OUTERWEAR

My personal experience showed that it is nice to have two pieces: an elegant one and a casual. I had a long coat and a bomber jacket. They did not go well with each other. If you are an ardent minimalist, you can get a thin jacket and an overcoat (so they would look good together) and not worry about any other outerwear. It all depends on your personal situation, of course, and the weather. You can add a trench coat, so that it would play the elegant role and the thin jacket would play the casual one when you move from summer to fall.

This is just a suggestion. I am well aware that everyone's situation is different. I am simply suggesting that you use the "business/casual/semi-formal/romantic" logic.

BOTTOMS

Follow the same principle here. Pick two or three bottoms of different cut that would work for all possible situations. For example, you can have business trousers, a skirt of suit fabric and jeans, where would we be without them!

Make sure the trousers are your type; they may be straight, flared, 7/8, culottes, or pipestem. Similarly, jeans and skirts ought to work for you personally. There are universal favorites, such as Bermuda shorts, culottes or midi skirts. They work well in both formal and informal situations.

TOPS (first layer)

I am going to repeat myself, like a broken record, "business /casual/semi-formal/romantic"

One of the tops ought to be semi-formal. It may be a silk blouse/shirt, a lingerie-style top or a top made of metalized knitwear.

Knitted tops, tees, long-sleeved, polo, and body tops all work. If you have two tees, I suggest that they should be on the opposite ends of contrast: a beige and a navy one, for example, or a black and a white one.

A sweatshirt or knitted jumper with a smooth texture works too.

You can use something knitted with yarn. It may be a sweater or a pullover with a neckline that works for you.

SHIRTS

I've put these into a separate category because they can work either as a first or a second layer. It doesn't really matter; it just depends on your life style.

You'll need one cotton shirt in the color that matches your color palette.

You'll also need one long and relaxed shirt that can be made either of cotton, denim or eco-leather. It can be used as a second layer or simply worn in various ways as the first layer.

TOPS (second layer)

There are two of them, according to the same "formal and informal" logic.

There is a jacket as the formal one.

And there is a cardigan, a soft relaxed jacket, or a thick shirt as the informal one.

ONE-PIECE

That's optional.

This would be a dress, a jumpsuit, or a jacket-and-pants set (that you already have). None of these items should be difficult to put together. They just need the footwear and accessories.

The dress should be a flowing one (lingerie-style would work too) that could be used with different second layers.

BAGS

You should have one primary one. It may be a stiff basic backpack bag or a small/medium basic bag.

You'll need one small one to go out.

You'll also need a relaxed bag, like a shopping one, a larger backpack, or a cross body bag.

FOOTWEAR

I don't think I'll list all of it. Just follow the same logic "formal, casual, semi-formal."

Here I will leave you and let you get back to working on your closet.

Chapter Seventeen
Step#14 How to Part with Clothes

You have already done so much!

You already have ideas for your capsule wardrobe.

I hope that in the meantime you are wearing and trying out things that landed in the 'maybe' category. You've rediscovered a couple of forgotten sweaters, hurray! You moved them to the 'favorites' category. But something else may be disturbing you. It's a sure sign that it's time to give it away.

You may be all set to give up the brown cardigan without a qualm, but there is still a pile of things that you're not ready to say good bye to. They are good clothes, but they won't work in the capsule. What do you do with them?

Here you've got to divide the leftovers into two parts.

The first category is for things you think you'll reactivate. Clothes that you like and that fit you well but won't work in this capsule either by color, or by lack of something to wear with them, or both. I suggest that you create other capsules for such things in the future.

LET'S SHOP IN OUR OWN CLOSET

The second category is for things that for whatever reason you do not wear and do not intend to revive. Oftentimes, these things are finicky and expensive.

There is also another category of expensive things, the ones that don't treat you well: the shoes chafe, the blouse twists, and the coat has a brand name but is awfully uncomfortable.

It's hard to part with them? I know just how you feel! I've been through it. I've done my share of emotional shopping. When you end up with creative and beautiful clothes, but all you feel is pity and guilt. You don't look any better in them (they buck and kick and won't work with you), but you feel bad about throwing them out; after all, you paid good money for them. And so, your closet gradually turns into a mausoleum.

It is very difficult to keep track of yourself. For example, it took me a while to realize that I am not a huge fan of scarves, although I've always thought just the opposite. Three-four scarves, including summer ones, is my optimistic maximum. However, I have a box full of scarves. They didn't all get there in a day, but that does not really change things. I've stopped trying to attack them like a bull with a red rag, but I still catch myself eyeing that box.

Here's another example. I used to hem my pants for the tallest heels. Why? I hardly ever wear heels. The same happened with jackets, I really practically never wear them. Especially in winter, under a coat – never, ever.

We get stuck in our habits and keep going on autopilot. Don't you think that our wardrobe is a goldmine for psychotherapists? The wardrobe so clearly demonstrates the mechanical nature of our habits.

I won't even say anything about sales and cheap clothes. You shouldn't shop for clothes as you would for hotdogs and ketchup. After all, how euphoric do you get over going grocery shopping?

There's another situation: a designer piece at an eighty percent discount. It's got a little defect but it's so tiny compared to the discount! Later on, because it was originally defective, it smoothly moves into the mausoleum category.

There is also shopping for the unreal you. For the one who is slimmer, more amusing, the one who goes hiking up a mountain three times a week, or the one who, it seems, is a society girl or a theater-lover. I am a dreamer, what about you? I agree, sometimes a dream, that is, a truly beautiful piece of clothing can really lead you on and change your life.

Are you having a really hard time parting with these?

There may be two reasons for it. The first is that we are stuck to our past like gum that's stuck to the paving. Do you know how long the suits from my past corporate life stayed in my closet? It's better if you don't. Is there a past you still knocking around in your closet, by any chance? Give her a big hug and let her go. If you want to keep a memory of her, take a photo and then let her go.

The second reason is fear of shortage. This needs a separate book. I won't delve any deeper here. There are reliable books and trainings on clearing space, letting go, friendship with your negative emotions, and so on. Here are two ideas I can give you.

The first one is related to money. How much does it cost to rent a square foot where you live? If you do not have problems with free space, then my argument is unlikely to work, but just add up the feet, calculate how much space your bankrupt clothes take, and how much you pay for things that do not give you any joy. Are you ready to pay that much, even if it's only a few dollars a months?

The second idea is also related to money, to your energy. We all invest in emotions. When you go to a beauty parlor, you may not become any more beautiful, but you're certainly poorer. Then you go to a movie, snuggle into a chair and exhale two hours later, having become richer in adrenaline and poorer by a certain amount of money. Giving away clothes is also an epic emotion. It means freedom, space and growth. It means giving yourself an incredible gift! You can make a ritual of it. Say, "Let all that needs to go, go." After all, people give away money for target marketing, red wine, or skydiving. You're giving away clothes. When push comes to shove, you've already spent the money.

Good luck!

Chapter Eighteen

Step #15 Conclusion and Some Reflections about Styles

The idea behind a capsule wardrobe is the absence of doubles or extras. It means the minimal number of pieces of clothing for various situations in life (I suggested four domains, but this is no dictate cut in stone). The point is the multifunctional use of clothes, the compatibility of clothes with each other, and a well thought-out color strategy.

The foundation of a capsule is clothes and accessories that we attribute to the Basics category.

To tame such an animal as a basic wardrobe and to put together a self-regulating capsule is an enormous achievement. Most people simply dress in basics and that's more than enough. Emma Watson, Katie Holmes, Jennifer Aniston, and many other beautiful women demonstrate the charms of a basic wardrobe.

Yet, many may want more than that. I don't mean more pieces of clothing, but more style-forming clothes.

No one said that you cannot introduce clothes of a more sophisticated cut or texture. For example, the domain I defined as semi-formal can include unique or original clothes and non-basic accessories.

How do we introduce more sophisticated clothes?

Let's assume that you have a jeans-and-jersey base. Let's introduce several pieces on the same theme. Let's start with a simple exercise. We'll just play with color, adding basic clothes of another color. For example, you feel like diversifying your wardrobe with an orange-yellow.

Then, every time you put together a look, you can add any number of clothes in the peach-and-pineapple palette. The minimum is two pieces.

For example, you can add socks and a scarf, or a skirt and hat, or shoes and a shawl. Two pieces of clothing should talk to each other, like accomplices; they should create a theme, set the style. It takes two to tango. This way, you'll give the word to one more of your sub-personalities, one happily full of vitamin C.

You can cite not only color that way, but also texture, prints or geometry in your look.

Let's make this a little more complicated. This time, you want to add not just color, but some romance. It works the same way. Add any number of items with a romantic-style attitude.

But you need at least two items in every look: a pink top and a pair of shoes, a delicate purse and a scarf. Are you tired of romance? Let's go military: military-style pants and a backpack, rough boots and a jacket.

Mixing basic clothes with style-forming ones is one of the most popular principles used in creating a look.

What do you need to know to introduce style-forming clothes?

You need to master the language of a particular style. Many speak the language of clothes intuitively, but I will try to set forth some key rules.

You can figure out what style a particular piece of clothing belongs to by these features:

Fabric

Color

Cut

Decorations

Mood

It is a very object-oriented study similar to studying grammar or vocabulary of a language.

There are some excellent Oxford foreign language textbooks, but, alas, there is no textbook on the language of styles.

I am not talking about fashion history. I mean a specific, practical present-day glossary; the kind that any normal woman, who did not graduate from the Antwerp Royal Fine Arts Academy, can use.

So that any woman could take a style text book, skim through it for half an hour, then open her laptop, go to an online shop and buy some clothes or accessories in a safari or marine style and quickly put together a very stylish and, what is most important, very up-to-date look.

What is the language of the basics? It encompasses neutrality, universality, and simplicity of cut (with no sophisticated necklines, slashes or tucks), compatibility with other clothes, and absence of sophisticated decorations, such as fringes, chains, rivets, or other accessories. They may be made of practically any fabrics, including leather. The color strategy may also be any at all, as long as it fits your taste. A basic wardrobe is an infinite game field and all brands give you a choice.

Can the same piece of clothing belong to several styles? Yes, including the basics.

We have approached a vast subject of styles that truly deserves a separate discussion. Reading articles and books on history of a particular style is a wonderful pastime, but it has never helped me. Back when I tried it, I was totally lost.

Even more muddle is created by the would-be styles. The so-called Street Style, for example. It is no style at all; it is bloggers who take pictures on the street. They are dressed stylishly, but there are no general consistent patterns in the looks they create. The only thing they have in common is pictures taken on the street. Or take the Oversized Style. That is no style either, they are just clothes cut in a certain way. Total Red, Total Any Color or Color Blocking are not styles either. They are color characteristics. There are quite a lot of such pseudo-styles. If you add historical lines to them, such as Victorian, in which costume designers are keenly interested, the muddle in your head gets even worse.

I am going to surprise you now.

Well, maybe not all of you.

You are already using many styles of clothing. You can't even imagine how many of them there are. You just do it, without even realizing it. Sometimes, that is precisely the reason why you cannot put together a particular look. It may be that your wardrobe is overflowing because you have collected a hodgepodge of things in it without realizing it.

I will tell you about popularly used modern styles and principles of creating looks in these styles in my future books. I hope to meet you there again. In the meantime, let's deal with the basic wardrobe and your first capsule. It is the most difficult and important step in taming a wardrobe.

Chapter Nineteen

Finding your Style

"What is my style?" many agonize over the question. In this part I will discuss just that and I hope you will find it helpful. I'll also talk about colors in more detail.

We are all different.

There are stylists who lead us to our goal, just like Goodwin, the Great and Terrible. We withdraw into ourselves; we take tests and put together mood boards and collages. We recognize ourselves in mythical characters and ask ourselves, "Am I a Moira or a Shahrazad?" After a long trek through the Emerald City, we buy a pink top.

There are stylists for whom an instant is enough. They do not ask us to follow the yellow-brick road, taking Lion, Scarecrow, and Tinman with us. They pick a pink top for us very quickly and, sometimes, without saying a word.

And then, there are women who buy a pink top without ever suspecting that someone had taken thousands of tests to make that decision and someone else has paid a lot of money to a personal shopper.

All roads work. Personally, I prefer the archetypical theory of color that I will tell you about in the chapter on color types.

These days, there are a lot of stylists who name themselves 'in-depth'. It seems to me that any movement towards yourself is just that – going into the depth. Even if you spend hours, picking out a suit for yourself, comparing prices, composition, and colors and then it all fizzles out. No luck. Because looking at it online is one thing, but here at home, when you put it on, it's something entirely different.

What can I say? Welcome to the deepest depths. Until you see the whole picture, you think that you'll never ever be stylish. You sigh, "It's all about money." But after all, you did not learn Italian in three weeks, one webinar, or even in a three-month class. Relax: learning the language of clothes is just like learning Italian, there is no end to it. I did have hopes. For yet another top that would put an end to my dressing struggles. Then I relaxed: this is how it's going to be and learning this language is so interesting.

Allow yourself to make mistakes and not be glamorous! All methods work: inside-out, outside-in, or in any direction at all. It does not matter which room you start with when you clean your house. Any move towards yourself is a deep one.

Chapter Twenty

How to Find Your Style "Inside-Out"

What are the ways to define a style? There are whole trainings built around the topic. I'll tell you about several ways and you can try the ones you like.

There are visual, projective tests. Tell me what type of flower you are, and I'll tell you who you are; tell me what picture you are and I'll tell you what color type you have; tell me what your ideal house is like and I'll tell you what you should wear. The simplest and most straightforward is to define a so-called style icon and adapt key style ideas to your appearance and budget. For example, you might like how Emma Watson dresses and her 'girl next door' looks. You feel akin to that style and you draw inspiration for new looks when you look at her. Or, maybe, you feel that you are the same type as Jennifer Lawrence. Everyone tells you so. And so you keep glancing at a woman who looks like you to see how she may wear something or other.

There are also psychological tests: NLP personality; Jung's archetypes; socionics, human design, and on and on. I'd get tired listing them all – there are thousands of tests. You can take any psychological concept you believe in and build an original class on style around it, something like "Inside-Out."

These tests are similar to the Cheshire cat – now it's there and now it's not. However complicated a description of your personality may be – Aphrodite combined with Demeter plus a bit of Hecate – it can be boiled down to the mischievous Cheshire cat's smile and a few words. Reduce that to three-five words and you get a verbal style statement. Then you can translate it into the language of clothes. And what is the language of clothes? It is color, texture, silhouette, and print!

Here is an exercise for you to illustrate the point. Ask your friends or relatives to give you feedback of several words that would describe you. Pick three words out of the results that make your heart sing. For example, they call you 'organized'. I wouldn't lift a finger with that description. But does *your* heart applaud it? If it does, take it, if not, move on to the next word. Did you find the three words that make your heart dance? Now it's time to bring them to life.

If you were called 'reliable', that is most likely how you dress too. Are you 'passionate' and 'fearless'? You are probably wearing elements that demonstrate that. It is a matching technic. You match, for example, your romantic side with romantic elements in your outfits.

A few years ago I read a book on defining two key words in the so-called style declaration. My two words are 'essential' and 'exotic' which, when translated into simple language, just means a muffin with icing. It's easy to picture what a simple muffin wears. To me pants and a sweatshirt (without sugar roses or coconut shavings) is a fantastically exciting outfit.

The language of clothes is universal, yet diverse. A single word can be represented by a thousand images. There are four billion women on the planet and that means there are four billion Aphrodites. All of us are goddesses of love, at least sometimes. My Aphrodite is very different from yours, yet we all recognize her. There are universal keys that everyone adapts to their look.

Unfortunately, no one teaches visual codes and languages at school. Nonetheless, we have all mastered these to a greater or lesser degree. You have to agree that your clothes speak even if you are silent. It is in your power to manage what they say about you.

There is an excellent book about visual perception by Malcolm Gladwell called *Blink: The Power of Thinking Without Thinking*. After all, it only takes us a few seconds to realize by looking at the sagging jeans whether we are dealing with a thug or a safe passerby. These few seconds promise no accuracy: you might discover a fake piece of art or win a war, but you might also lose millions of dollars or even kill someone. But in these high-speed times, you often need to understand or figure out who you are dealing with in just that handful of seconds. On average, we see hundreds more people a day than we did a hundred years ago. It is up to us to manage the impression we create.

You can see how words are interpreted in clothes in certain movies. I would recommend several episodes of *Once Upon a Time*. It's all about an evil witch cursing the entire fairy-tale world. The characters of parables, fables and fairy stories end up in the early 21st century in a town where time stopped. Why do I recommend this particular movie? Fairy tale characters are archetypical: the Queen is evil, Belle of *Beauty and the Beast* is the embodiment of beauty and femininity, Snow White is everyone's favorite princess, Emma (Snow White's daughter) is the savior and Little Red Riding Hood is a misfit on the fringes of society. Watch how the fairy tale characters are dressed in modern clothes and what a wonderful translation the costume designers have made.

Chapter Twenty-One
How to Find your style "Ouside-In"

There are those who start with appearance, who go from outside to the inside. For example, there is a famous theory developed by Grace Margaret Morton and Harriet Tilden McJimsey *. Later on, it was borrowed and adapted and now it is known as the Kibbe Theory. Morton studied nature from the point of view of yang and yin energy and ways to express it.

Where are you on the Yin and Yang scale?

Picture the coordinate axes. Zero marks the Classic point. This is where beauty combines the square and the round, Yin and Yang in equal proportion. On the one side of the Classic are the more feminine types (Romantic, Juvenile, and Angel) – those who have a lot of S and O lines. On the other side are those who have more yang in their appearance (Dramatic, Athletic, better known as Natural, and Gamine). They have a lot of L and Z lines. The classification was somewhat modified by Kibbe, but the key idea is still the same.

There are clear-cut types, but mostly, we are a symphony of archetypes. I have a bit more of the Yang. I recognized myself in the Dramatic who never grew up, that is in Gamine, as well as in Classic and a little bit in the Natural type.

What type are you?

The idea behind the Morton and McJimsey theory is that a certain style is inherent to each type.

Let's take the Angels, for example. They are tall – remember the elves in The Lord of the Rings. They have narrow, elongated figures. Look at ballerinas and models. There is something mystic and unearthly in them; they walk as if floating in the air. They look ageless. They like light fabrics, such as chiffon and light knitting; tie-die, and iridescence. They gravitate towards clothes where the structure is not obvious – tunics, skirts with asymmetric hem, palazzo trousers. They go with layers, fluidity, and feathers. Their timeless clothing has a vintage effect.

Or let's take, for example, the Classic. Why even talk about it? We all know what classical beauty is. Balance is its second name. Since they balance between Yin and Yang, the end result is conservative – neither short nor long, neither wide nor narrow. They are elegant and proportional in their repeated silhouettes. They may be chic, but never unique or super sophisticated. Imagine the style of present-day princesses who cannot do without protocol.

I am sure you get the idea. If you are interested in learning more, read Morton and McJimsey.

For those of you who do not want to tie yourself into a pretzel, who do not like introspection, those who wonder "What do I do with all these archetypes and personalities?" and who have no energy for a stylist, but simply want the suit to fit nicely, go back – all the way to the chapter on "How to Find Your Individual Style while Staying Right by Your Closet."

Here is a piece of summing-up advice. There are two categories of people. Some don't like to have boundaries and limitations and others do. And that is wonderful! I can really understand those who simply couldn't care less about all these theories on style search. Any guidelines are restrictive and get in their way of making a choice that is not easy to begin with. Others, on the other hand, like self-reflection, tests and help in focusing. From my point of you, joy should be the key criterion. Does knowing that you have a 'Natural' type of appearance help or hinder you?

Chapter Twenty-Two
Suzanne Caygill's Seasonal Color Analysis

Suzanne Caygill came up with the Archetypical Theory of Seasonal Color Analysis early in the 20th century. Unfortunately, she has removed all the text from her only book, so there is no point in buying it. Her legacy, however, is still alive. It is supported and developed by a group of her fans in California.

As we learned in our Physics classes, color is wave energy. Suzanne Caygill said, "Color Is the Essence of You," and that says it all. Suzanne studied colors using the perfection of nature. She found keys in it to our color and designer templates. Beauty is defined not by size, style, color or build, but rather by the vibration that exists in every human being. Suzanne calls this vibration the essence of the person. When clothes and colors are the extension of us, this essence becomes more apparent – we brighten up. That is when people tell you how nice you look, how rested, how slim and glowing. People notice you, instead of your dress or your shoes.

The Archetypical Theory of Seasonal Color Analysis is not just about what colors look good on you; it is about how you appear in space. It is about your energy that manifests in the tone of your voice, your walk, and the lines of your body. It is about where you work well, where you rest well, and even about marketing that is native to you.

The theory broadcasts one of my key values – ENERGY that we can all do with more of. When you are in your color, you are in yourself. You have to agree that we are always looking for what belongs to us. After all, how is the color palette built? Half of the colors are you: the color of your eyes, skin, your cheeks, veins, and the whites of your eyes. The other half is a bit more creative: it includes your accents, metals, and pastels.

Naturally, after reading my short notes, you are not likely to become an expert. But you don't need to. I would like you to be interested in color and be aware of it. Next time you go shopping, put things up to your face, think about them, play with them.

Chapter Twenty-Three
Winter Color Type

Esthetically speaking, I am quite urban. That means that a city suits me from the stylistic point of view – all those polished surfaces and patterned Portuguese tiles.

Some people are suited best to savannas, others to 18th century mansions; I am best suited to a modern city.

Ask me, where I look good.

The answer is – in a Japanese restaurant. There, everything is wintry: the sushi, the tableware, the interior design, and myself in winter colors. Not because I am Asian; Coco Chanel in a little black dress would look good there too. So would Jackie Kennedy in her kimono-like suits.

Imagine that such a very urban person goes to the country. Nothing there is as it should be: the lighting is different, everything is eclectic, there is lots of greenery, and lots and lots of texture.

What happened to me? An existential crisis. I didn't just change the landscape. I exchanged the corporate jail-like environment for so-called freedom. I suddenly became the mom of a seven-year-old. Everything changed at once.

The Japanese (a culture with very wintery esthetics) would say that I lost face. It took me a long time to paint a new one. Dress-wise, I went down to the depths of hell – to shapeless knitwear.

Back then, the idea that wearing something loose and shapeless can be turned to my advantage never came to my mind. Put everything in the same range of colors; not even complimentary colors, simply various hues of the same color – hoodies, pants, coat. Sing an ode to monochrome and you'll turn into a feminine, inky goddess just like the one on Chinese wrappers? Not on your life! Go for wabi-sabi or shibumi? Whatever is that? What goddess? I was drowning in my own hesitation, permanent soul-searching, and knitwear.

I had to do something about the existential crisis. My search began with style. Now, don't think me a stylish gal. I'm as far away from stylish as the bottom of the deepest pit is from the surface of the Earth. Venus is my planet and my karma. I like things to be functional and, if possible, pretty. Heels don't usually make it.

I told you that it doesn't matter which room you pick to start house-cleaning. I started with a deserted guest house. It may not have been the best decision strategically. If I were to start over, I'd go to a big-time shrink and glue my face back on. But my karma called me.

What is the Winter archetype?

It is Contrast and Depth.

Look at Chanel, she was Winter and whatever she created is just a continuation of what she is. I cannot imagine Chanel creating anything frivolous, with frills and cheerful flowers.

I also have an undying love for black and white. I am black-and-white. Despite the fact that many are loud in saying that we should leave off black, I will stay faithful to this combination that is inherent to Winters. Chanel left her legacy of the little black dress for Winters and for some Springs.

A few years ago I watched short video interviews with women fashion designers. There were offices and break-rooms in the video too. Vera Wang, whose color type is Winter, takes her breaks in an absolutely empty, bare room. She is fed and nourished by such surroundings. There were two orchids on the window sills and she thought even they were too much.

Winters usually love universal emptiness and that love is true not only for monochrome clothing, but also for their self-expression through interior or website design. Universal emptiness does not necessary mean naked, hospital-like walls. Winters love unique accents, like the ones in a snowy landscape: an abstract print on a tee-shirt, a bright necklace, a section of a red wall in an interior.

The contrast inherent in Winters is their mission on Earth. Men with the Winter color type are either heroes or bandits. Winters need to shock their public and if they don't do it by their appearance, they do it by public speaking or mentoring. They make good leaders, editors, and critics. They can stand back. Let's say that you are a modest-looking Winter, such as me, then your tendency to stand out will express itself in your creative work. My *femme fatale* manifests herself in this book. How about other examples? Let's take Diana Vreeland with her key value of uniqueness or Steve Jobs – no comments needed there.

Winter colors are all about hardship, danger and beauty. I don't need to tell you about winter landscapes. A pure archetype would have alabaster skin and dark hair. I've a friend like that. If she puts on a red necklace, everyone is enthralled. Winters can wear contrasts without being lost behind them. On the contrary, they disappear or look dull in more muted colors.

The winter pink is fuchsia. The green is a rich emerald. The blue is indigo, sapphire or ultramarine. The white is as iridescent as fresh snow.

The purple and its derivatives is an intense orchid. Black – you can't really do without it! Diamonds and all cool glittering gems are their best friends.

They look good in business, classical, and dramatic clothes.

Who makes clothes for them? Chanel, Dior, and the minimalists.

Here are good descriptive words for Winters:

- Regal

- Absolute

- Deep

- Exact

- Pure

- Contrasting

- Perfect

- Dangerous

- Austere

They might even use some of these words when they speak.

You would be right to ask, "There are eight billion people on the planet. Do they all come into just four categories?"

There are all types of energy in us. In some people one of the types dominates, others are borderline types. Some may be warm-cool, with hazel eyes, for example, and a cool undertone to their skin; some may be just the other way around. Add to that your culture, climate, temperament, and experience. All palettes are quite individual, but there are patterns.

Chapter Twenty-Four
Spring and Summer Color Types

There used to be a time when I went to pick up my daughter from school with a double purpose: I wanted to get my daughter and look at two of the teachers.

One of them was the Spring color type, the other one was the Summer.

Spring was double-lucky: first she had the color type and second – her figure type was an inverted triangle.

I went there for inspiration. You could have taken pictures of the Spring teacher every day and posted them on Instagram. Her pearlized slip-ons went so well with her hair color, the knitted tops hung so beautifully on her wide shoulders, and there was a scarf around her neck too! The milky colors looked so good on her. She had the most difficult age group – two and a half and up and, despite her workload, she was and still is the best-dressed teacher in the school.

I haven't seen what's known as the 'effortless style' very often. Every case of it was a Spring or, occasionally, a Winter (well, it's easy for Winters to understand themselves). It's not because Springs and Winters are born with clothes-sense. Not at all. It is simply easier for them to figure out their appearance and it's easier for them to live as consumers – everything that's sold these days is for them. Bright prints and whitened colors don't make for rocket science. Besides, salespeople need to attract the customers' attention. What colors and prints are the most resonant and catchy?

What is Spring?

Spring is champagne. It's Hollywood. It's the tang of a spring breeze. They are pretty, sexy, and very yin. If they are not pretty and yin, like that teacher was, then they are athletic. They may sometimes be a bit rough. They are extraverted. There are some introverts, but they are either pretending or have convinced themselves somewhere deep down. They are sometimes annoyingly energetic. They keep flapping their wings tirelessly, like a hummingbird. I know what I am talking about. My husband, his sisters, and several friends are all of the Spring color type. I am surrounded by Springers.

Men and children love them. Instagram loves them too. They live in bright, catchy colors, just like children's cartoons. And all of it is effortless. They are better at going live than at writing texts. If they do write, energy bursts forth from their texts. We all want them, like champagne. You wouldn't happen to pretend to be a Spring? Don't bother.

What else? Mozart and Van Gough.

Lots of designers make their clothes, starting with Stella McCartney and all the way to Benetton.

Spring is not a story about Winter's perfection, but about blooming, energy, and Easter eggs.

If you watch the spring awakening in nature, you will see all spring colors, starting with the delicate snowdrops and all the way to the riot of tulips. This freshness of color comes when you dilute the pure pigment with water or add white. Springs are water-colors.

Their blue is the blue of the bright sky or turquoise. The green is apples and grapes. Red is the ripening cherries. Disney Land with its cotton candy, confetti, and soda pop is also a Spring-themed park.

There are as many Spring subtypes as there are flowers in a meadow. Despite all this diversity, they all share their youthfulness and the direction of energy from inside out.

They are not complicated or tenacious. They flare up, have a screaming fit, and keep going to charge-annoy you with their energy. They like simplicity. All of this is demonstrated in their style, accessories, and interior design. They go for simple understandable forms that are sometimes even childish. Their clothes are of fresh bright colors but simple cuts. The simple, slightly athletic style was created for many of them. The champagne energy often comes through in liking glitter, something shiny, sweaters with beads or sequins.

Here are some descriptive words that fit Springs:

- Energetic
- Pure
- Happy
- Sunny
- Bright
- Bouncy
- Light
- Vibrant
- Radiant

***

Now, let's talk about the Summer color type. The Summer teacher was the most beautiful. It's not just my personal opinion; compliments came from other parents too. But she did not sparkle. She had a hard time. Her body was feminine, beautiful. Jeans (either straight or skinny) and oxfords didn't make her size 8 any slimmer. It would have been nice to see her in a dress and a veiled hat.

Summers are the women you don't notice at first. But once you do see them, you can't take your eyes off them. They are beautiful, sophisticated, and introverted. When I say introverted, I don't meet closed-up. Many Summer girls, would be indignant, "I am not an introvert! I've so many friends and contacts!" But we are talking more about energy types. You may have thousands of subscribers, friends and acquaintances. Or you may even be a public person. But your energy is still smooth. Summer is not a fountain or a geyser; it is a smoothly flowing river.

The words enchanting and mesmerizing were created to describe Summer women. Simply by their presence, they pull us into a calming world and you never even suspect that you have already drowned. How many times have I melted in their hypnotic softness? There I would be, the Snow Queen, and suddenly, it's not me but just one large puddle. How do they do it? They just sit quietly, without taking a grandstand like the other color types do.

These milk-and-water girls only look soft and delicate; actually, they are strong and powerful, just like the river that flooded my house. Actresses of the Spring color type, for example, are not flexible at all. Yes, they are fun and funny and pretty, but that's all. They usually play parts that are very similar. Summer actresses can play anything.

If we talk about appearances, they look like they are covered in mist. It's as if they were here from the old days that can never come back. It is easy to picture them wearing something long, elegant and flowing. Vintage mansions, silks, and cashmere suit them better than anyone else.

For Winters, symmetry is inherent. Their essence can be shown as parallel lines. For Springs it is a circle, stars, and hearts. Summer women are more about slight curves. Their geometry is about the oval and the letter S. One of my Summer-colored friends says that she experiences unspeakable delight when drawing the treble clef.

Summer women, just like Winters, have a cool skin undertone. But their story is not about contrast at all. Their intricate powdered colors speak of finesse, calmness, and sophistication. They dress enchantingly and mesmerizingly. They wear prints about melancholy and the riddle of the labyrinth. All in all, they draw you in. You have to pause and take a closer look. If they wear flowers, they'll be bottomless Fibonacci roses or something well-tended, not a spring meadow. They love details. Lots of small details.

Their red is a dried rose, a strawberry, or pink quartz. Their blue is a Douglas fir. The green is seafoam. White may be like the inside of a shell. Many of them wear pearls remarkably well.

Who makes their clothes? Try looking up Brunello Cucinelli.

Descriptions:

- Delicate

- Flowing

- Soft

- Beautiful

- Gentle

- Elegant

- Sophisticated

- Aristocratic

- Misty

Have you recognized yourself in any of the color types? You think about it and in the meantime, I'll tell you about the Fall color type.

Chapter Twenty-Five
Fall Color Type

I looked for women with an expressed Fall color type for a long time. It seemed to me that they didn't range in my habitat. Then I saw them. One was in my Dutch class and the other was among the parents in the school yard.

They both looked like wild animals. One looked like a lynx and the other like a chestnut-colored wild horse. I admired them. They were so unusual. Asphalt didn't suit them. They looked alien in our plastic civilization. I was too shy to ask them about their ancestry. They were both white, European women. Where did they get that particular skin tone from?

It is easy to picture such women in a hunting lodge reclining on animal skins; or by the campfire in a desert, dressed in military or safari style. I could just hear the drums and the rumble of earth. If they land in an office for some reason, they make everyone run, not just stroll. I had a boss like that once. Johnny Depp would be the height of phlegmatic next to him. One of the Fall-colored ladies I mentioned above said of herself, "I have such a temper that I am always mad at something."

Fall is the season of transformation and abundance of fruit. There is something in the women of the Fall color type that is just as active and unpredictable as the fall weather.

If you imagine a corporation, the right distribution of labor would look like this: Spring attracts clients and is responsible for sales and marketing; Summer takes care of the books, HR, and operations in general; Fall gets the projects moving: they do not walk, they run dragging the rest with them; and Winter manages all this.

If you compare the Archetypical Theory of Color with the famous Hippocratic Bodily Humours theory developed by Galen, this is what you get:

Detached Atos – Winter

Cheerful Portos - Spring

Soft Aramis – Summer

D'Artagnan who keeps the plot going – Fall.

Remember, early in the book I promised to tell you why I divided our life and our wardrobe into four domains (casual, business, romantic and semi-formal)?

Fall is about presence, heyday, maturity, and celebration.

Winter is about business style, professionalism, and detachment.

Spring is casual; it's about the joy of creation and sports.

Summer is about being with people; it's about love and romance.

But let's go back to the Falls.

Safari, leopard prints, wind-blown fall leaves, and flames, they are, all of them, for women of the Fall color type who are active, wild, and sensual. There is a bit of angularity, awkwardness, or danger of the wild beast in them. Fall is not like the parallel lines of Winter, it is more like a zigzag. What else goes with them? The baroque, the richness of Venetian glasswork, the gaiety of carnivals, gold and brocade. The more texture the better. The famous saying that "less is more" was certainly not made by a Fall.

Their red is pomegranate, brick, or burnt sienna. Blue is a peacock's breast or the warm sea blue. Their palette has all the richness of fall leaves. The colors are not pure, they are sophisticated. They are often made by adding a pure brown pigment.

Who makes their clothes? Dries Van Noten, for example.

Words that describe Falls:

- Dynamic

- Luxurious

- Metallic

- Spicy

- Rich

- Strong

- Copper

- Flaming

- Mature

Chapter Twenty-Six

On branding and color palette

In this chapter, I am going to tell you what colors make up your color palette, how to use it, and what role colors play in your life.

It is just a concept, and it is not mandatory, of course. But I believe that honey can be gathered from any flower even if the flower seems unattractive.

Let us say that you have nothing to do with the stage, that you are not a Fashion freak, not an emo or a punk, and that you don't have any particular role. Your goal is to let your natural beauty shine, while exerting as little effort as possible. It would be nice if people understood all about you without a cover letter or long-winded explanations. Besides, you don't have a lot of time. All this sounds just like my life: get breakfast quickly, drop the kid off at school, listen to my husband's words of wisdom, oh, and find out what's on with targeting and marketing. Whether you want it or not, you strive for energy, for support of your appearance at the color level.

Oh and then, there is the subject of branding that everyone is so tired of. Here, I am going to suggest an infallible point of view. Look at yourself as a patch of color. Lose your shape and spread out like the clocks of Salvador Dali or like eggs in a pan. Of the palette you get (you, when you are spread out), take certain colors and paint your website, Instagram, and home with them. Your heart wants to show itself as color. Are you a psychologist? Paint your office walls in nude, to spread the exposure all around you.

I'll tell you how it works in more details below.

So what do we have?

The color of your irises, the whites of your eyes, your skin tone and hair color, the color of your veins and blush. There are so many colors inherent in us. Let's talk about the sacred triangle.

WE WILL START WITH YOUR EYES – LET'S WEAR THEM!

Let's say that you work with people, in HR, for example. You want to keep the person you talk to in focus, to broadcast the message "I am easy to talk to." We are not talking about looking venerable or dazing them, so they forget what you're talking about. You want the person you are talking to to look directly into the mirror of your heart.

To do that, you have to wear your eyes. That means, wear clothes that match your eye color. The effect is heightened if you combine it with your white, in other words, the whites of the eyes are added to the color of irises. Picture a white scarf with a drop of a grey-blue that spreads out into the white space. The deepest color is the iris, and the white space is for the whites of the eyes (this is for the blue-eyed beauties, if you have eyes of another color, the drop will, naturally, be a different color too).

When you wear clothes the color of your eyes, you express balance. It's the color that's like the center board on a sailboat or the middle note on a piano. It's the balancing point on a seesaw. You are balanced and can be sensitive to others. If you look at your eyes carefully, you will find numerous facets that make up the light of your eyes. When you wear these colors you truly inspire yourself and others.

Wearing the color of your eyes is not a burden energy-wise. Usually, they are not very bright colors. You have to try to find the shades that make your eyes brighter and not duller.

SKIN TONE OR COLOR NUDE

Let's say you need to draw someone out. If you want people to feel relaxed and open to discussing intimate questions with you, become intimate – meet them in the nude.

What is intimate? It is something very personal, very heartfelt. It is a very close link or a deep understanding of a place or a person.

Your skin tone expresses closeness, a connection, a kinship. Wear clothes of that color when you want to improve confidence or start a relationship. Wear that color if you want to be extremely open and sincere. It is good for family reunions, first dates, or meetings with children. It's a perfect color for bedrooms and family rooms.

I read that some professionals paint their office walls 'their beige' as if extending themselves to their walls. According to them, the effect on the clients was immediate. The nude color makes us a bit vulnerable; it expresses our basic essence, after all, it is our second skin. It is not as absolute and isolating as black. When we wear it, we feel calm and elegant. Try it. If you already have clothes like that, feel how different your sensations are when you wear them.

The list of skin tones is quite large: from alabaster to dark chocolate. Besides, there are people who have 'simple' skin, without undertones and there are those whose skin is 'complex'. I am telling you this, so that you realize just how many shades of beige or nude there are. I would like to inspire you to find your own. If you have already found your foundation tone, you can use it as your template.

HAIR COLOR

Let's talk about the largest and most important accessory to our appearance – our hair.

Since we are talking about colors, we are not going to discuss shapes or styles. Take a close look at your hair color. It is not even, it consists of highlights and lighter and darker shades. Pick out colors that would be the 'ambassadors' of your hair color and bear in mind that you don't need an exact match. Don't get stuck with just the one color either. Remember that color appears differently in different textures. Come up with several options.

What do you do with this information?

Buy clothes in that color. You might buy overcoats, sweaters or dresses in your hair color. In most cases, this color creates a casual effect and, most importantly, it harmonizes the entire look.

You can repeat your hair color in your look. For example, you might want to use accessories in your hair color: a bag, a belt, or shoes.

Your hair gives you an idea of texture that you can use in your clothes and in your furnishings, for example. Curly hair has a coarser texture and you can repeat it in coarse netting or a mohair sweater quite excitingly.

So, we found three important colors. If your blog is about sincerity and psychology, take the color of your eyes, skin, and hair as your primary theme. Are you doing a podcast or a selling post? Then add a couple of accents. Do you want to broadcast love? Add your shade of red. You have to be careful when you pick your colors here. For example, if your red is wine, it is best not to pick a brick-red. See below for more on reds and other colors.

OTHER COLORS OF YOUR PALETTE

Pink stands for the feminine principle and the survival of the species. It is the color of sexuality. It highlights and amplifies femininity in women and masculinity in men.

Let's try to define your pink. Look at the palms of your hands and your face. It is the color that is close to a natural blush. You can use your blush makeup as a template.

You blush when you pinch your skin, go for a jog, or are nervous before a date with your prince. It's your heartbeat, the pulse of red blood that you can see through your skin. It is your life force expressed by hemoglobin. It's the color of conviction, danger, and courage. When you wear red, you are emotionally convincing and can express your passion.

Red may vary from pink to coral, form the color of rust to a bright red or pink.

What's your black? If there is no black in your appearance, you can use the darkest shade of your hair color or eye color. It's really simple.

What about white? The whites of your eyes, the white of your teeth.

We dress as ourselves. We literally create a second skin. We have found what is called neutral colors. It took me a long time to figure out what this animal was. Stylists give you various lists of neutral colors. It's irritating. It only became clear when I have found this particular explanation.

Let me tell you about myself: I am monochrome. It turns out that there is only one pigment in me. Sometimes it deepens to a dark brown, almost black in hair and eye color, sometimes it's diluted to olive skin and is completely absent from eye whites. So it comes down to a range from white to black. This monochrome is overlaid by bright colors, my accents. That's my presentation of myself. It's quite simple really.

What are you like?

All we have to do now is to find your accent colors.

To make it simple, we can say that the color of power or the accent color is determined by the choice of color that is the counterpart of red. Every color has its opposite on the color wheel. For example, a color contrasting red is green, just like black is the counterpart to white. If your romantic is a bright red, then your color of power may be a color in the bright green range. It is best to play with them and put them up to your face to see which shades empower you, which of them make you come alive and look brilliant.

The color of power is the most dramatic, the most eye-catching color in the palette. You should wear it when you want to be noticed. For example, wear it to a presentation. It is better to use the color of power to attract attention than black and white, especially if your personal palette does not have a pure black or a pure white. This color is the true representation of the most dynamic part of your personality. It's a palette based on studying nature and it is not likely that you can get a more powerful image than the one nature created.

There may be several accent colors.

Some type of blue, for example, suits everyone. We all have veins, after all. The question is which blue? In general, the color blue can express anything, starting with power and drama and all the way to reliability and serenity. When we add black to the blue, we get the harshness of winter; when the blue is diluted and whitened, it broadcasts purity and amusement. We need to play, experiment, and search.

There are also pastels and subdued colors. We might say they are of the "meet the mother-in-law" type. We use them when we want to tone down our presence. They are best used when you announce yourself to be a team player, as when you are a backing vocalist, for example.

This leaves prints. A print is your face. It has the same lines, contrast, and your colors.

Every time you buy new clothes, make sure you see what they look like on you in daylight. Clothes should pay you compliments. They should not switch you on, but they should amplify your inner light. Do you hear people say, "What a great dress, pants, shirt!"? That's your warning signal. Who was complimented – you or the dress? If you rush towards a certain color, ask yourself again in about ten minutes – you might change your mind.

Have you suddenly found that certain colors give you a surge of joy? Introduce them into your life a little at a time, so you can get used to the new and unsettling.

Remember the first capsule we've put together for a Kate Winslet type? We used the following colors: hair color (suit), her red (sweatshirt), eye color (blouse), her pink (skirt), skin color (the beige tee), her white in the shirt and accent colors in the shoes.

Chapter Twenty-Seven

Your expectations from the book

Many of you have picked up this book hoping to solve your personal stylistic problems. To hear something like this, said personally to you:

For example,

"Lisa, why do you need those white sneakers? Why this inappropriate contrast between the snowy white and the stout blue of the denim jacket? Don't you have a choice? Why not take lavender, olive, or dusty rose ones? You are not such a simple person. Leave the snow for the Springs and Winters."

Or, something like this,

"Jane, there is a type that Max Mara makes clothes for exclusively. I don't mean for you to go bankrupt, but why don't you browse through or go and try some on. You can then come up with something similar for yourself."

Or yet like this,

"Alice, your leading archetype is the Seeker, you're a strong businesswoman. Why push your Lover archetype on Instagram? Save it for your husband."

LET'S SHOP IN OUR OWN CLOSET

To list all stylistic practices in the world is equivalent to clearing all the sand in Sahara.

Downloading five hundred and sixty gigabytes of styles, as they downloaded Kung Fu into Neo's memory is just not possible.

TRUST ME!

Style is when practice comes before theory.

I remember how I used to sit down with a cup of fragrant tea to hear yet another lecture (not a luxury I can indulge in these days). It seemed to me afterwards that I grew smarter. My brain thought it had worked. But the solitude by the closet stayed with me. Why would you need dead knowledge?

I suggest that you become your own stylist.

Take two or three new things and try them out, think about them, try to get an insight. Celebrate your finds.

You will never be one hundred percent satisfied. You are always growing. And that's wonderful!

Here is my favorite quote about beauty by Milorad Pavic:

"Beauty is so difficult and so hard to create that when we come into contact with something beautiful, we feel relief, realizing that in the general distribution of energy in the world, we have been spared a certain amount of labor. Someone else's effort, invested in beauty, reduced our share of tiredness, released us from a certain expenditure of effort and that is why we can enjoy beauty. We simply rest in beauty..."

Let us give some rest to others, to your family, your clients, and random passersby.

I love champagne. I am raising my glass to you, my beautiful reader! To you!

With love,

A.A.

Thank you

Thank you very much for reading the book. I would love to hear your thoughts. Your feedback will help me to improve my following books. Would be grateful if you could leave your review or write to me: alayaaifel@gmail.com